Feed, Burp, Change, Repeat
Conquering Your Twin Journey

A comprehensive guide to what lies ahead on your twin journey with special sections on marriage and intimacy to strengthen your marriage bond, and a custom diet and exercise section to help you get rid of that twin belly.

Feed, Burp, Change, Repeat…Life with a newborn has its moments. Life with twin newborns has triple. Moments with one baby, moments with the second baby, and precious moments the twins share together.
It took 38 weeks before my twin girls moved out of my body and into the world. 38 weeks, 35 doctors appointments, 22 sonograms, 18 blood pressure scares, 17 weeks of monotonous bed rest, and 8 false alarm trips to the hospital. My hormones raged like a fierce river throughout the entire pregnancy. My swelling was worse than it had ever been. I was so sick I thought I would never be able to eat again. And I couldn't breathe. My body was NOT my own. It was being held hostage by those two little lives…

But out of that trial, birthed the most amazing experience I've ever had. Twins. They are the light of my life. And the reason I wrote this book.

You see I have experience with children, and lots of it. I have 8 children, ranging in age from 21 years old to infant. 4 boys, 4 girls. I've been raising children in a quickly changing/evolving society. What worked for my first-born will not work for my last. Parenting has become one of the greatest challenges I face. Yet out of the trials and tribulations that come with having 8 children, I've learned so much. And I'd like to share that knowledge with you. This is not just a survival guide for twins it is a guide that can help anyone who is pregnant. I haven't held anything back. I wanted to deliver a comprehensive guide that you could use to help you survive parenting for two. And if you are parenting for one baby, it will work for you too!

I hope you can read through the sections of this book with your partner so you catch a glimpse of what you both can expect...and what each other is going through. As difficult as it was for me, it was just as difficult for my husband. Sometimes we can get so wrapped up in our own world that we forget how much what we go through affects others. So please read this book together. I believe it will help you grow and bring you closer. It will take BOTH of you to get through the next several months. Both of you.

Whether you are pregnant with twins, or have already birthed the bundles of joy, this book is for you. So that you can sit back and have confidence that you can do it. And enjoy the precious moments with your twins that you will never get to re-live.

CHAPTER ONE
Surviving the weirdness
Being pregnant with twins and the body complications you may face.

If you hadn't noticed already, being pregnant with twins is a TOTALLY different ballgame; a ballgame that you enter into without much training and help from the outside world. Most of the information about pregnancy that is on the Internet is about single pregnancies...called singletons. That's a word I read a lot while I was pregnant with my two. The information available about being pregnant with twins is scarce. I didn't think my doctors knew a lot either although they were making double and triple the money from my twin pregnancy. It was very discouraging. However, after I searched I discovered a few websites that had some information. There was one in particular that I read during my pregnancy. This website even had pictures of a twin pregnancy belly.

I browsed through the illustrations in an attempt to arm myself with what was to come. The twin belly pictures ended at 36 weeks. And if you compared the single pregnancy pictures with the twin pregnancy pictures it was enough to scare anyone. That twin pregnancy belly was HUGE. HUGE. Way bigger than the singleton.

I tried to find comfort in knowing I would be full term at 36 or 37 weeks, that's when most experts agree (and by the way there aren't really any experts about twin pregnancy) the babies are ready to be born. I also read that 1/3 of twins are born early BEFORE 36 weeks. Certainly the odds were in my favor that I would not reach the size of that 36 weeks twin pregnancy belly. Which I found comfort in because I didn't think my body could stretch that big. Boy was I wrong. I went to 39 grueling weeks. And my belly did get that big!

I had been pregnant several times before the twins. I birthed 6 children prior to this pregnancy. All of them were birthed vaginally and I was able to have them with virtually nothing to block the pain during labor. I was a self-proclaimed expert on childbirth. I went to a birthing center for one birth. Another baby came into the world when it was just he and I, locked in the bathroom in pain. Yep, I delivered my own baby. Surely I could handle a pregnancy with two. Right? Easy!

NOT. I really thought I was going to die. With every new week came a new challenge for my body and mind. I was so sick, so tired, and so moody. My marriage was on shaky ground, I lost close friends, and my parenting was a nightmare with all the extra stress I had. I was miserable. And I was making everyone around me miserable too.

The first several weeks of my twin pregnancy, I was so sick that my husband would get a kick out of saying, "maybe there's two in there." He would tell me this after I finished throwing my guts up in the bathroom. I couldn't keep anything down. I had never had morning sickness before. But this wasn't even morning sickness. It was afternoon and evening sickness too. And it was terrible.

Then my friend Donna said the same thing. "Maybe you're having twins." She agreed that I had never been this sick with any of my previous pregnancies.

Our pastor counseled my husband and I and he called us DOUBLY FRUITFUL. He kept saying it over and over again. Apparently God was trying to tell us something…but I didn't want to listen. I wanted everyone to stop. It wasn't funny. I thought they were all crazy. So I kept everything I could of my pregnant free lifestyle to set out and prove them wrong. No one in my family had spontaneous twins. My cousin had In-vitro fertilization and 2 of her 3 eggs took and she had twins…but spontaneous (naturally conceived) twins just did not run in my family. I kept my workout regimen, I ran a 10K race with my son, I kept coaching basketball, and I stayed at school full time for my senior year in college. I had no idea that what was happening inside of me was going to slowly tear me down.

"Are you sure about your dates?" The nurse asked as she firmly pressed on my belly. I had finally made it to my first doctor's appointment with the pregnancy.

"Yes. I am sure." I remembered the night like it was yesterday. I knew exactly how far along I was. And exactly when I'd had my last period.

"Let me bring you to ultrasound. Your uterus seems like you are further along than you think. I want to get the dates right." I hate it when people don't believe me. They make me feel like I'm an idiot. I began to protest but figured I'd let her measure and she'd find out I was right. At least that's what I expected would happen.

On my way to the ultrasound room I motioned my husband to follow us. He was patiently waiting in the hallway and was happy when he found out we were going to get a glimpse at the baby. For him, this was his first experience with pregnancy. I had been a single mom of 6 kids for 5 years patiently waiting on my prince. And along he came, my husband Bill. He was quite a special man to take on all I had and then deal with a newly pregnant wife. I sometimes wondered if I was going to break him. But so far so good ☺.

"Is it twins?" He asked the nurse. Bill smiled. I gave him the 'you are in trouble' look. We went into the dark ultrasound room, I positioned myself on the table, and the nurse located the baby and began to take measurements.

Several minutes went by as they were looking at the baby on the display. I saw one baby on the screen, it was very tiny but I could see it. I called out to my husband, "see…only one baby in there." And that's when it happened. No sooner did I mutter that sentence and let it hang in the air for a moment when the nurse shook her head and answered me a quiet "no."

She continued. "No, there are two in there. I'm going to get the doctor just to be sure." And with that, she left the room.

WHAT??? I looked over at my husband. He looked back at me. We were in shock. Well, I was in shock and he was in heaven because he was right. *Twins. Two babies? How the heck were we going to afford two babies?* The nurse came back into the room with the doctor, who verified there were two babies brewing deep inside. I looked at the screen as they pointed out their location to my husband and me. I felt like I was going to throw up.

Apparently I was the only one in the room who didn't find it amazing that I was pregnant with twins. Everyone else was rejoicing. The entire staff at the doctor's office was rejoicing. I was fighting back my breakfast. We left the office that day, pictures in hand, and went to lunch to let the news sink in. I was still in utter shock. And I couldn't eat.

What should've been the happiest moments of my life, I lived in utter shock and despair. I didn't know any truth to what I was going to go through and I was frightened. I did not enjoy my pregnancy with two. Do not be like me and do what I did. Sit back, relax, and read through this entire book. Over and over again if you want to. Arm yourself with the information you seek and realize that you are going to be okay and that with a little planning, this pregnancy can be successful and you can have two healthy babies to hold in your arms very soon. Take a big deep breath and relax. It's going to be okay.

So what should you expect when you are expecting two? What does it feel like? Will you run out of room? Will you be able to walk towards the last few months? Will you be able to breathe? How can you survive the seemingly un-survivable? I am gong to answer those burning questions for you...

I am not going to break it down week by week and inform you of what to expect while carrying two. There are too many unknowns with a single pregnancy but when you are pregnant with twins, those unknowns multiply 100 fold. Instead, I'm going to break it up into categories and summarize what you should expect or at least prepare for and hope it doesn't happen to you!

Sickness

I had never experienced morning sickness during any of my previous 6 pregnancies. Morning sickness with the twins was totally new to me. And it was rough.

They say one of the first signs that indicate you may be carrying multiples is when you experience morning sickness on steroids. Lovely, huh? Thanks to extra babies we experience mega hormones. Our bodies have a hard time adjusting to these new hormone levels and so our stomachs are under attack. If you don't get sickness, that is great. But being pregnant with multiples virtually GUARANTEES you will experience it at some point in your pregnancy. So what causes it anyways? And is there a way to ease the suffering? There are three main causes of morning sickness...

- **Hormones from H**L:** During pregnancy, your lovely hormone levels increase rapidly. These levels skyrocket to prepare your body for the upcoming pregnancy challenges that lie ahead. These rising hormone levels are the first culprit in triggering nausea and vomiting. Unfortunately when you are pregnant with twins these levels are even higher which means more nausea and vomiting for you!

- **Your new SUPERNOSE:** You will be super sensitive to smells this pregnancy. Again, it's the lovely increasing hormone levels in your body that cause this. Some of your most favorite foods might make you run to the bathroom now so beware and be prepared to bolt like a superhero!

- **The Hostile Takeover of your GI Tract:** During pregnancy, your GI tract also becomes extremely sensitive. It slows down, fills with bloating and gas, and is soooo uncooperative. Food takes longer to digest, and longer time in your GI means more irritation. My stomach was not my own when I was pregnant. The additional hormone levels in pregnancy slow down the activity of smooth muscle tissue for a good reason. It actually helps your body absorb extra nutrients for your unborn child. With two babies it slows down even more so that more nutrients can be absorbed. And there is nothing you can do to stop it.

But fear no evil from your stomach…here are some helpful tips to help you get through the hostile takeover of your digestion…some might work some might not.

- Eat small meals and snacks frequently throughout the day. HAHA if you can stand to eat. An empty stomach can trigger nausea. The suggestion is eating every two to three hours but this never helped me. Because I simply couldn't eat.

- Protect your sniffer. Stay away from strong smells and if you smell them…RUN!!! Try not to cook strong-smelling foods and if you do consider cooking them outside…I'M SERIOUS. I had to kick out the deep fryer while I was pregnant. It made me so sick. Even the smell of the oil when it wasn't being used was enough to send me running to the bathroom. The deep fryer was removed from the kitchen, placed in the garage and remained there until after the twins were born. Actually it's still there now but after my husband reads this I'm sure he will remember the deep fryer and be reunited with it.

- Keep plain crackers by your bedside. Eat them before your feet hit the floor in the morning. This helped stave off my first bout of sickness. And it really works. Later in the day crackers didn't do so well for me.

- Drink water. Fluids will help you from getting dehydrated and will soothe the stomach. OKAY…whatever. Everything made me sick, even water. But you might benefit from some extra hydration so try it and find out if it helps. My goal was to get 8 glasses in daily. But I had to sometimes chew on ice cubes to help stave off nausea. Sucking or chewing on ice cubes is better than nothing. Make a water goal for your day and stick to it.

- Avoid fatty foods and spicy foods. These foods are hard for your stomach to digest and may trigger nausea and vomiting. ACTUALLY I had to hang up the healthy diet and I found fatty foods helped my stomach.

Everyone is different. What works for one person may or may not work for you. Try the above tips and if you find any that work that aren't listed, send me an email or blog. I will add it to the book to help others get through. But sickness will go away. And I found the only permanent solution was to deliver the babies. Today I feel great. My stomach is still a little bit sensitive but I have returned to normal eating again.

Exhaustion

There isn't enough caffeine in the world to give pregnant women the energy they need. When I was pregnant with my twins this couldn't be more accurate. Energy is at an all time low as your body is trying to accommodate for the two new lives developing inside. Your body literally steals your energy to grow your babies. Making matters worse, while you are pregnant you should LIMIT your caffeine intake to protect your babies. So how do you do this and keep the energy you need to get through the day? UMMM…Miracle please. You need a miracle.

When I was pregnant with the twins I was tired. I was tired going to my car. I was tired taking the kids to school. I was tired in college classes as I was listening to the professors lecture, I was tired cooking and cleaning.

When I was coaching basketball, I had to sit in a chair and yell to the kids…because I was so tired. I didn't want to walk up and down the stairs because I was tired. I was so tired that I couldn't even fall asleep some days after I laid down in bed…it was just too exhausting! How can you get more energy to help you make it through the exhausting day?

Of course, you know the first piece of advice I'm going to give here. Get plenty of sleep. Sleep is the most important thing you can do for your body while you are pregnant. It is rough on your body to carry twins. Sleep is what your body needs to replenish all the systems and repair all the cells that you've used damaged during the day. If you don't get adequate sleep you just spin yourself in a downward energy-sapping spiral.

As you get further along, you will find it harder to sleep. So try to get as much sleep in the beginning as possible because it will get more uncomfortable as the months drag on. Like an animal stores food for the winter when food is scarce, you will need to store sleep for the last trimester when sleep is almost non-existent.

First, try to get more sleep at night.

1. Set up a REGULAR bedtime. Going to sleep at the same time every night will help you train your body to settle down and shut down.
2. Set up a REGULAR wake time. As important as it is to go to sleep at the same time every night, it's equally important to wake up at the same time every morning.
3. Nap regularly to make up for lost sleep. Sometimes my best sleep was in the middle of the day when everyone in my home was away. Use down time to your advantage and catch up on some zzzzs.

4.   Do not go to sleep right after dinner. Sometimes you will feel very drowsy after you've eaten dinner. Fight sleeping at this time because chances are you will wake up and not be able to fall back asleep again for several hours.

Second, eliminate caffeine. If you must have a small pick me up, choose to drink your stimulating beverage as early as possible in the day. And limit that cup of Joe to about 50mg caffeine. It is not the time in your life to become a regular consumer of espresso or latte. Opt for regular coffee and keep it in a small cup. If you have to, pour the rest of the pot out or purchase a single cup coffee maker.

Third, naturally regulate your sleep-wake cycles. This means exposure to light during the day, and limited exposure to light at night. During the evening turn down the lights in the house, turn off the computers, and limit television viewing. During the day open the blinds and keep light pouring in.

Fourth, stay away from large meals at night. This is pretty easy when you can't eat anything anyways.

Fifth, get regular exercise. As long as your doctor hasn't put you on movement limits, try to get some form of regular daily exercise. This could be a brisk walk, slow jog, or exercise on a stationary machine. Now is NOT the time to ride your bike or roller-blade outdoors. Before getting pregnant with the twins, I rode my bicycle about 60 miles every week. While I was pregnant I had to hang my helmet up and quit outdoor cycling entirely. You need to keep your feet on solid ground when you are pregnant because a fall can hurt your babies and you. It's temporary so don't worry. Safety is important.

Sixth, keep stress and anxiety away day and night. HAHA HAHA…yes, I'm laughing. This is a joke. When I was pregnant I was so stressed out. My hormones made me a monster. I was worried and depressed and anxious all at the same time. Stress seemed to be my middle name. So how can you stress less when it seems like stress is overtaking you? I've consulted some experts and added some extra tips myself that may help you stress less, as you are falling asleep when stress hits you at its hardest. This is not the time in your life to be superwoman ☺.

1. Get out of your head. Have you ever noticed how you can go through your entire day and not think about things that are bothering you, but when you lay down to sleep at night the entire list starts running through your head? This is because during the day you are distracted. So try to distract your head at night by listening to soft music, utilizing some deep breathing exercises, and thinking about only calm positive things when you lay down.

2. Turn off the television and read a book. I used to fall asleep reading my textbooks or the Bible. I could not read a magazine or an exciting novel because these simply turned my brain on. So I chose to read something that wasn't too stimulating for my brain. When I was younger I used to fall asleep reading my school textbooks all the time. Since I was still in college when I was pregnant with my twins, I brought my textbooks in my bedroom and read away. It took about five minutes before my face was firmly planted in the pages and I was sleeping away. I always wondered if it was possible to absorb the information through the skin in my face, but it never happened that way.

3. Escape. You need to find a way to relax, even in the middle of chaos happening all around you. This is a great tip you should try to perfect before the babies come. With a houseful of kids, there are plenty of opportunities during the day to yell and run around like the hulk. My boys are active. They also have very different

personalities. So fighting is a daily occurrence in my home. I have learned to take baths, pray in a corner, walk outside and sit on the front porch for a few minutes, or go upstairs to lock myself in the room. You must find a way to escape-I call it my time-out. But especially after the twins are born and you can't seem to get away for even one second, you must train yourself to relax and escape in the middle of all the chaos.

4. Lean on your husband. Literally. Snuggle up into his chest or shoulder area and let the zzzs overtake you. Sensing physical touch is a great way to help you relax. Everyone needs physical touch. EVERYONE. So don't feel like you're being silly when you ask your husband to help in this area. You can't ask him to take over the pregnancy so it's the least he can do to help.

5. Have sex. This goes without saying but I still had to mention it here. Sex is a really good way to let go of stress and afterwards drift peacefully away to sleep. Sex can be very taxing on your body, especially later at night. Make sure you have regular times with your husband so that you can not only continue the wonderful bond that the two of you have, but you can also catch some much needed sleep.

And finally, make your bedroom sleep-friendly. This means keep your noise levels down, keep the temperature right, and keep your bed comfy. Noise levels in your bedroom need to be kept low. If your husband likes to watch television and browse the internet when you are trying to get some zzzs, kick him out of the room or ask him to limit those times to when you aren't lying next to him trying to fall asleep.

The optimal temperature for sleep is around 65 degrees Fahrenheit. Although I couldn't keep my room that cold, I did keep it cooler at night than I kept it during the day. Research has proven that a cool room leads to a better night's sleep. We kept ours around 72 during the overnight and that seems to be a good temperature for us.

Make sure your bed is comfortable. We actually had to buy a new bed during my pregnancy. I was not comfortable at all in our old one. Unfortunately the new bed wasn't much better but I did get more sleep on it. After I recovered from childbirth I realized my new bed was very comfortable. If you are in your third trimester you might not find any bed in the world comfortable enough for you to get a good night's sleep. So don't go out and impulsively buy an expensive bed. From 27 weeks on I spent most nights tossing and turning in the living room on our couch. Sleep is just not fun at the end of a twin pregnancy.

Swelling

My legs were so swollen when I was pregnant with the twins. I elevated my feet often to try to get rid of some of the water retention. I avoided salt and caffeine. But nothing I did seemed to alleviate the swelling. I was miserable and looked it! My shoe size went up 1½ sizes. My feet were so ugly with the extra swelling and it was difficult to walk. Sometimes my lower legs would go numb from the added pressure.

This swelling I experienced was actually "typical" as my doctor said for twin pregnancy. Most swelling during pregnancy is normal and perfectly safe. All women experience some amount of water retention when they are pregnant. Also when you are pregnant fluid shifts to tissues inside your body adding to the edema (swelling).

Why do you swell? Your quickly expanding uterus puts pressure on your pelvic veins and your vena cava (the large vein located on the right side of your body that carries blood from your lower limbs back to the heart). This increased pressure slows the return of blood from your legs, causing it to pool, which forces fluid to remain in your veins in the tissues of your feet and ankles. The result? Swollen ankles and feet.

This swelling is more prominent in the last trimester however I noticed the increased swelling in the beginning of my 5th month. Being pregnant with twins just causes so much more stuff than pregnancy with singletons! But before you explode like a water balloon, there are some things you can do to help alleviate the swelling.

- Put your lower legs and feet up whenever possible. At home, make the recliner your best friend. At work, keep a stool under your desk. This does help but as soon as you get up and get mobile, the swelling seems to return to your legs.

- Don't cross your legs or ankles. Keep them safely apart whether you are standing around or sitting. I did this…it didn't help.

- Keep a good supply of blood flowing to your lower half. You can stretch your legs while sitting and see if this helps. Or you can flex your foot to stretch out your overtaxed leg muscles. And of course movement at the ankle can help too. I used to draw the alphabet in the air with my foot to improve my circulation. You can try this and see if it works for you.

- Take regular breaks from sitting or standing. Experts suggest a short walk every so often because it will help keep blood from pooling in your lower extremities. If you are on bed rest this will not be able to be done.

- Choose your footwear wisely. Pick out comfortable shoes that stretch to accommodate any swelling in your feet. Heels are a no-no unless the pump isn't very high. Think comfort NOT fashion.

- Avoid the temptation to wear socks or stockings that have tight bands around the ankles or calves. When I used to wear socks for the day, there was so much swelling from the sock line up especially at the ankle that the difference would remain for hours despite my desperate attempts to elevate my feet and alleviate the swelling.

- Many people suggest wearing waist-high maternity support stockings. I live in Florida so I couldn't wear stockings while I was pregnant. But if you choose to wear them, put them on before you get out of bed in the morning. This way fluid doesn't have a chance to pool around your ankles.

- Drink plenty of water. No matter how many times you have to rush to the bathroom dehydration is the biggest culprit in swelling. Because you are pregnant with twins your hydration needs go up. Drinking extra water will help alleviate swelling.

- Get moving. Regular exercise such as walking, swimming, or stationary bike riding will help move water around inside your body and may help reduce swelling. Again, if you are on bed rest this cannot be done.

- Avoid junk food. Especially high salt foods like French fries. As good as they taste right now they are really bad for your water retention. Avoid high salt foods entirely while you are pregnant. This will also help reduce your blood pressure.

If you don't' think swelling is that big of a deal think again. While I was recovering from my c-section, they had to rush me back in the hospital for hypertensive crisis because there was so much excess fluid in my body that it caused my already high blood pressure (Pregnancy induced hypertension) to soar to critical levels. I didn't realize how bad the swelling was until the hospital informed me that for my short 4 day stay I had lost over 12 pounds of fluid because of the meds they had given me to flush the fluid out. WOW.

Weird Skin things

It has been over 11 months since I had my twins and I'm still battling with weird skin things. I never had skin tags or this "line of pregnancy" with any other birth. And to still have these issues 11 months later is very discouraging. Your skin will change so much during your twin pregnancy. And unfortunately there's nothing you can do to prevent skin changes. Just keep hydrated and lay off the lotions unless your skin is really dry. Choose hypoallergenic lotions and make sure you uncover your skin and let it breathe once in a while. Once your hormone levels return to "normal", these skin things should go away. I'm still waiting on mine to leave but my hormones are still a little off right now.

Here is a list of 10 funky skin conditions you might experience while pregnant with two. There are more but I listed the most common ones. If something strange shows up on your skin ask your doctor. If you are like me and need to figure it out on your own, search it on the Internet, look at pictures, but still ask your doctor after you've made your diagnosis.

1. The "pregnancy glow." You are glowing now. Really. An increased supply of blood you are experiencing as a result of your 'babies on board' causes your cheeks to take on a blush color. Your oil glands secrete more oil and this creates a nice sheen for your skin. The results? A glowing complexion!

2. The pregnancy mask. Brownish or yellowish patches called chloasma (dubbed the mask of pregnancy) may appear sometime around your second trimester. Hormones are once again the cause of this condition. The pregnancy mask can appear anywhere on the face but are most commonly detected on the upper cheeks, nose, forehead, and chin. Estrogen and progesterone are to blame (imagine that, hormones again). These hormones stimulate the melanin cells in the skin to produce extra pigment, but in blotchy patches. There is no way to prevent these but if you limit your exposure to sunlight and other ultraviolet light it will reduce the appearance.

3. Linea nigra. Many women normally have a white line running from their navel to the center of their pubic bone. It is faint and barely visible before pregnancy. Sometime in the second trimester when it's getting hard to move around, you may be surprised because your linea alba becomes a linea nigra, a dark line that is more noticeable. In some women the line extends upward from the navel as well. The linea nigra disappears several months after delivery. I never had one in the six pregnancies prior to my twin delivery. With my twins, it appeared and four months postpartum it is still fading.

4. Acne. Zits, zits, and more zits. Are you serious? I don't ever have a problem with acne but when I was pregnant with my twins, it showed up. Just treat your skin gently if these problem pimples appear. Avoid using abrasive cleansers, scrubs, or exfoliates. Wash your face twice a day. And opt for oatmeal-based facial products. You cannot use prescription drugs for acne while you are pregnant because of the risk of birth defects.

5. Dark areas become darker. Little moles and freckles that existed prior to pregnancy may now become bigger, and brown spots or birthmarks become browner. New moles may also appear. (Consult your doctor or dermatologist if these moles seem particularly raised, dark, or have irregular borders.) The areola and nipples of your breasts will become quite a lot darker; unlike other areas of your skin, which return to their original color after pregnancy, your areola will probably always be somewhat darker than they were before you were pregnant.

6. Spider veins. Your circulatory system is on OVERLOAD. Increased pregnancy hormones and increased blood volume cause tiny and squiggly red or purple lines to appear just below the surface of your skin. These are capillaries. These spider veins (named this because they resemble a web) pop out in the face or on the white part of the eyeballs during the delivery. The downside of this weird skin condition is that spider veins may not go away after pregnancy. A dermatologist can remove them postpartum by using injections.

7. Heat rash. Your body during this time might be hotter than normal. An overheated pregnant body mixed with excess perspiration and the friction of skin rubbing can lead to prickly pimply irritating heat rash. Limit your time in the sun and outdoors if it is summer and when indoors cool off by sipping on ice water and taking a cool shower.

8. Skin tags. Ugh. I suffer from these to this day. Apparently you are more prone to tiny polyps, called skin tags, appearing in areas where skin rubs on clothing or the skin rubs together. Most often these are found under the arms, between neck folds, under bra lines, or on the inner thighs. Skin tags are a result of a hyperactive growth of a superficial layer of skin. Supposedly they disappear several months after delivery but mine are still hanging around.

9. Itching. I itched SO BAD when I was pregnant with my twins. I itched everywhere on my body. From head to toe. I itched really badly after six months gestation because my skin was stretching and these areas are more prone to feeling itchy. All I can tell you here is scratch scratch scratch. But be careful not to irritate the skin further.

10. Pimply eruptions. Less common than ALL The other skin conditions, itchy and red patches may appear on your stomach, thighs, buttocks, arms, and legs. This condition has a nickname-PUPP. It's actually called pruritic urticarial papules and plaques of pregnancy. It appears during the second half of pregnancy and disappears shortly after delivery.

Hair

Today I am mourning the loss of my pregnancy hair. I had lustrous and beautiful locks throughout my pregnancy. This is due to less shedding of your hair during pregnancy. Normally 90% of your hair is in a growing phase while 10% enters a resting phase. Every 2-3 months the resting hair falls out, allowing new hair to grow in its place. During pregnancy more hair enters the resting phase but does not fall out until after pregnancy. Your body holds onto your hair and you will notice less hair falling out or coming out in your hairbrush. Unfortunately, just like all the other changes, this is temporary. Eventually your body will shed off the excess hair it's accumulated during pregnancy and your locks will return to their pre-pregnancy condition.

Expect this hair loss, because half of all pregnant women experience it. It begins about 3 months after delivery but should taper off before 5 months postpartum. Sometimes it keeps shedding and shedding. Don't freak out. That hair that's coming out at a record rate is actually hair that should've fallen out months ago. It's not extra hair loss; it's delayed hair loss. Try to clean the drains in the sinks and showers more often so the delayed hair loss doesn't create a bigger plumbing problem down the road.

But during pregnancy enjoy the luxurious locks. I took the opportunity to grow my hair longer during my pregnancy. I stopped going to my hair appointments and let my hair grow only trimming it one time during the entire pregnancy. I'm glad I did because I realized I don't need my hair cut as often as I get it cut which saves money and time when you have neither once those babies are born.

The jury's still out on the safety of perms, hair color, and bleach during pregnancy. My advice here is to use wisdom. Limit your exposure to these chemicals. Opt for a more natural hair dye that is less abrasive to your skin. Curl your hair with curlers instead of getting a perm. During my pregnancy I still dyed my hair. I have some sections of grey hair and needed to cover them up. But I did get a touch up type stick to use between colorings so I could color my hair less often. And I learned how to hide the grey roots by styling my hair differently.

Iron levels in blood

This is where I'm going to get real frank with you. I hate taking Iron pills. Hate it hate it hate it. Also, because my prenatal vitamins had extra Iron in them I hated taking those too. I need to have regular bowel movements daily. It is just a thing I have. If I don't have at least one movement a day I freak out. So Iron was NOT MY FRIEND during pregnancy. In fact, it was the enemy.

After I had the babies I reaped what I sowed with my lack of Iron. My Iron levels plummeted. They gave me extra Iron in the hospital and stool softeners to help me go. It just didn't help. It was almost too late. So I suffered for the first 6 weeks postpartum with Iron levels around 6.5. Complicating that was my pregnancy-induced hypertension that I was heavily medicated for. I felt like absolute crap. My hair turned white...half of it went completely white most likely from the iron deficiency. And if I had to do it all over again, I would've take the Iron pills and eaten extra salad to help move things through.

You must take your iron. Every day. And with twins you need extra iron. Talk to your doctor about a good iron supplement to take while you are pregnant. To help you with your constipation, I've listed several foods that you can try so that you can remain regular throughout your pregnancy. Just remember that your digestion is much slower now. And if all else fails and it's been a few days since your last movement, talk to your doctor. But don't stop taking the Iron pills and don't self-medicate with stool softeners. It might be harmful to you and your babies.

FOODS THAT MAKE YOU MOVE ☺

It's all about fiber. I know you hear it all the time. Fiber fiber fiber. But did you know that fiber not only regulates your digestion, it actually creates resistance for your intestines that makes your digestive system stronger? It's like lifting weights for your intestines. Fiber not only helps over the long haul it helps during your pregnancy to help get things moving. So fiber up! 25-30 grams daily. Here are some foods rich in fiber that you can eat to help you add punch to your poop and guide you on your road to regularity (yes, I totally had fun with that sentence).

Veggies: Vegetables rich in fiber include; broccoli, kale squash, sweet potatoes, pumpkin, collard greens, and leafy salad greens. Okay, so that list is totally yucky to the pregnant woman. But fear not, several other food groups contain fiber-rich food.

Fruits: Both fresh and dried fruits are helpful to your movement mission. Fruits with peels like apples, pears, and oranges are great choices. Also blackberries, blueberries, plums, peaches, and grapes can help get things going. Of course if all else fails, opt for the ultimate movement makers-these include dates, figs, prunes, and raisins.

Grains: Whenever you choose your carbohydrates with your meal, have fiber on your mind. Opt for whole grains instead of refined sugars. Use wheat bread instead of white, whole-wheat pasta instead of regular, brown rice instead of white rice and oatmeal instead of regular cereal. There are some high-fiber cereals on the market that you can try as well. I always kept a bran cereal near by and placed it in a bowl to munch on when my tummy was growling. Read labels and choose the item with the greatest amount of fiber listed.

Beans. Okay…now this is risky. Because your digestion is SLOW gas is present in much greater amounts in your digestive tract. Try beans but only in small amounts. I personally couldn't eat beans while I was pregnant. It was painful. So don't be surprised if this is one food item you just can't have.

As important as it is so eat foods that will help move your digestion along, it is equally important to avoid the foods that can trigger constipation. I've listed the constipation culprits here. Try to avoid eating these items as they can cause more harm than good. Especially avoid them at night when your body slows down even further to get ready for sleep.

FOODS TO LIMIT FOR PREVENTING CONSTIPATION

1. Dairy -Although it's important to get extra calcium at this point in your life, dairy products can trigger constipation. If you are suffering from slow bowels, axe the dairy temporarily and get your calcium through a supplement. Just keep in mind that calcium and Iron supplements need to be taken at different times of the day, as these two tend to cancel each other out when taken together.
2. Low Fiber High Fat Frozen Dinners-These quick to cook meals slow down your system. Low fiber high fat foods set the pace for your digestive tract at SLOW. Because fat slows digestion down, avoid any foods that are high in fat. At this point you need all the help you can get and that means abstaining from slow movers like fat.
3. Cookies-Cookies are low in fluid, normally high in refined sugars, and contain fats. They slow down your go. Avoid them and opt for some fresh fruit instead.
4. Bananas-Bananas can be bad. Depending on their ripeness. If you eat a green un-ripened banana it can

slow things down. However if you grab a nice ripe banana it can speed things up. Same food with much different results!

5. Fried foods-those yummy fries could be causing more damage than your think. Fat, greasy foods tend to slow movement through your digestive tract. Choose broiling or steaming foods instead. Stay away from fried...it's constipating and not very healthy for you or your babies.

Blood Pressure

It's time to discuss blood pressure. Personally, I've always had lower blood pressure readings. I have never had a high-pressure reading in my life. Whether I'm in pain, very sick, or nervous at the doctor's office, my blood pressure readings hold steady at 110/65. However, when I got pregnant with the twins and was placed on bed rest, things got crazy inside of my body, particularly with my blood pressures.

I was a very active person before I was placed on bed rest. My normal exercise routine involved distance running, distance biking, and weight training. I did something active every day, even when I was feeling under the weather. So when bed rest came upon me, I literally took every open and able blood vessel in my body and shut them tighter to accommodate the inactivity. The result? High blood pressure. My body simply didn't need all those highways and byways to run blood through anymore so it closed them down.

Towards the last trimester of my pregnancy, my blood pressure got worse. My readings were high and often the nurse would take my pressures, force me to sit calmly, and take the pressures again to see if they were any lower. I visited the doctor almost every week. So almost every week I had the same problem, high blood pressure.

They checked my urine for protein, and re-checked it. I went to the hospital so much to check the babies and help lower my blood pressure that my health insurance ran out and I was left with a $50,000.00 medical bill. It was a nightmare. Every week I went into the Labor and Delivery Unit. They all knew me well. We were on a first name basis with the staff. The hospital staff did several ultrasounds on the babies. I knew all the ultrasound technicians too. I was so sick of going to the hospital that I did everything in my power to lower my blood pressure. But it wasn't enough. And even after delivery I suffered for six weeks with high blood pressure readings. At one point I was on 600mg of Beta Blockers and 35mg of a Calcium Channel Blockers just to keep me at 145/90 B.P.! And this was all because I was pregnant with twins.

So what do you do? Listen to you doctor's advice, lower you stress levels, TRY to get sleep, and learn to relax. These will all help in reducing your risk for complications from high blood pressure. Don't follow in my footsteps on this one. Don't end up back in the hospital four days after the babies are born and end up fighting for your life. Stress kills…especially a new mom. If you want to survive you must learn how to stay calm.

Constipation

The same thing that causes nausea when food enters the body can also cause discomfort when waste tries to exit the body. Slower digestion doesn't end at your stomach; it is slower digestion all the way to the end. Constipation may be more common during your twin pregnancy. Eat more green, leafy vegetables if you can stand them, avoid excess dairy products that might aggravate an already slow system, and listen to your body.

Don't struggle to have a bowel movement. During pregnancy you are more prone to hemorrhoids (strained veins within the walls of the anus). I listed several foods in the section about Iron that you can use to help 'move things along'. Refer to it and if you find something that works better for you, use it. Remember no two bodies and no two pregnancies are exactly the same. I had 7 pregnancies and NONE of them were similar. Listen to your body and keep on top of your digestion. You will be feeling full enough at this point in your life. And constipation only complicates that feeling.

Breathing

While I was pregnant with my twins I couldn't breathe at all. The last 2 months of pregnancy were the worst. I would actually catch my breath sometimes because my breathing pattern was so out of whack. Some days I wondered if I would ever be able to breathe right again.

I can breathe now, but while I was pregnant oxygen felt like it was depleted in my system. Complicating matters was the fact that I am a distance runner and biker. My activity level overtaxed my entire body and left me gasping for air often. I was gasping for air so often that I had to quit working out entirely.

Lucky for you the breathing problem is due to yet another accommodation your body makes while taking care of those precious twin babies inside. And of course HORMONES are to blame ☺. The hormone progesterone stimulates the respiratory cells in the brain to ask for more oxygen and your body responds by meeting the greater demand. The pace of breathing does not increase, but the amount of air that goes in with each breath you take increases.

A pregnant woman can inhale up to 40% more air than usual with every breath. But it sure doesn't feel like more air does it? Unfortunately this breathlessness is around to stay until the babies drop before delivery and give you a little relief or until the babies are born.

There are 2 other causes of breathlessness during pregnancy.

1. Extra pressure your expanding uterus is placing on your diaphragm. When you inhale the diaphragm must pull down in order to accommodate the room necessary to allow the lungs to inflate with air. The pressure of the growing babies will crowd the diaphragm and make breathing labored.
2. Your blood is different. There is a higher level of carbon dioxide gas that is now circulating in your blood because of your pregnancy. This level increases because the growing baby inside must get rid of its own carbon dioxide gas (a waste product) and this is done through their umbilical cord, out the placenta, and into the woman to be expelled in the blood stream.

Although breathlessness is perfectly normal, if it will not go away, gets worse, or is accompanied by pain in the chest or upper back area as you breathe it is time to call your doctor. These pains are no joke and you must get medical attention to rule out any underlying heart or lung conditions.

If you are experiencing breathlessness (and I'm sure you are), there are some things you can do to get relief. First, you definitely need to slow down what you are doing when you feel your breathing become labored. Also, you should go to the nearest chair and sit down and push your shoulders behind to give more space for your lungs to inhale more air. This position also helps give more room to the diaphragm.

At night if you are experiencing breathlessness, a few pillows placed underneath your back so you can be propped up might also provide some relief.

Pain

With twin pregnancy comes many different aches and pains in numerous places around the body. You could experience a sudden sharp pain or the pain could last longer and be less severe. Pain is inevitable. I've narrowed down a list of pregnancy pains to the most common ones. If you have a pain not on the list don't worry. I probably could've listed about 200 different pains. This is only a list of the most frequent types.

The first three H pain symptoms…

HEADACHES

There are two main types of headaches you can experience while being pregnant. Unfortunately, there is no a lot you can do to prevent the headaches. The two types of headaches are tension headaches and the all too famous migraine headaches.

1. Tension headaches. Ouch! Ugh. I never had headaches until I was pregnant with twins. Unfortunately during pregnancy headaches are common. This sudden ache on both sides of your head is referred to as a tension headache. Hmm…tension. Think you have tension? Probably. Tension headaches are most likely due to the rush of hormones that your body is experiencing. And of course with twins those hormones are double! Other causes of tension headaches are fatigue, allergies, straining your eyes, stress, hunger, sinus congestion, and dehydration.

2. Migraines. Isn't lovely that about 15 percent of all migraine headaches occur for the first time for a woman while she is pregnant? Migraine headaches can last up to 72 hours! How do you know if it's a migraine or a tension headache? Tension headaches are usually located on both sides of the head while migraines tend to land themselves on one side only.

What can you do about it? Talk with your doctor. Acetaminophen is regarded as safe to take during pregnancy but only your doctor can make a specific recommendation. Drink plenty of water, eat protein, and reduce your stress levels to combat these nasty headaches. And of course, get plenty of rest!

HEARTBURN

Do you feel an awful burning sensation that comes up from your stomach and travels all the way up your throat? Do you try to eat food and drink fluids to quench this strange fire that seems to be taking over your body? Heartburn is the most awful side effect of pregnancy (I think) because it's with you every single day and it doesn't go away no matter how hard you try to get rid of it. Antacids don't seem to last more than 1 minute to stop heartburn. Changing positions while sleeping at times seems to just aggravate it. Stress you are feeling of course amplifies it. Heartburn, in summary, is no fun!

So what is heartburn? And why does it seem worse with your twin pregnancy? Heartburn (also called acid reflux or acid indigestion) is defined as a burning sensation that originates from the bottom of the breastbone and travels up to the throat. It's caused by those awesome hormonal and physical changes your body is going through. And unfortunately, heartburn won't go away until after the babies are born no matter how much you do to try to get rid of it.

And it's a condition that is once again caused by the placenta (the root of all physical evil in mom and the root of all nutrition and health for the babies). During the pregnancy the placenta is hard at work producing the hormone progesterone, which causes the smooth muscles of the uterus to relax. Unfortunately this hormone can't zone in on one section of smooth muscle tissue, so it signals ALL the smooth muscle tissue throughout your body to relax. One of these muscles effected by the hormone is a tiny valve that separates the esophagus from the stomach, thereby allowing all kinds of digestive juices (gastric acids) to travel back up towards the throat. Enter-Heartburn!

Progesterone (again?) also slows down the wavelike contractions inside your esophagus and intestines that help move food through your digestive system. So enter sluggish digestion combined with acid traveling back up---more heartburn!

Oh, and it gets better. Once the babies get to be a certain size (earlier for twin pregnancy but for singletons around the midpoint of the pregnancy) they crowd your abdominal cavity moving all kinds of important stuff out of the way and this pressure adds to heartburn by pushing the stomach acids back up into the esophagus. Pure awesomeness!

So what can you do about it? You can try a number of things to try to reduce the discomfort you are feeling as a result of your heartburn. I seriously tried almost everything and nothing ever worked. So again, this list is only a suggestion. Try the different methods and see what works for you.

1. Say no to the food that triggers heartburn. These foods include carbonated beverages, alcohol, caffeine, acidic foods like citrus fruits and fruit juices, tomatoes, mustard, vinegar, processed meats (which

you shouldn't have anyways), and of course spicy and high fat foods.

2. Eat small meals. Filling your stomach with less food will cause less acid to accumulate in your stomach and this will cause less acid to come back up towards your throat.

3. Don't drink a lot of water at meals. Instead get your 8 to 10 full glasses a day between meals.

4. Avoid eating food close to bedtime. Experts suggest eating at least two to three hours before you lay down for the night as gravity helps keep stomach acid down.

5. Sleep like a total weirdo. Prop yourself up with pillows or a wedge. This will also keep stomach acids down as gravity will pull the acid back in place.

6. Chew gum after you eat to help stimulate your salivary glands. Saliva helps neutralize stomach acid. But I must protest here because I'm a gum addict and chew it ALL the time. My heartburn never ever went away.

7. Wear loose clothing. Ha-ha what the heck else are you going to wear? Wow. Apparently tighter clothing helps push things back up too. But I just don't see the clothing having any kind of effect on heartburn when you have two babies in there fighting for room!

8. Don't smoke or drink. Well, that's a no brainer. But if you are to this point in my book and you are still struggling in this area, there are quit lines that you can call and get help. And talk to your doctor. Honesty is always the best policy. These babies only have one stay in your body...you need to make that stay as safe as possible by avoiding smoking and drinking.

If none of these measures work, talk to your doctor/caregiver about medications that he/she can prescribe to help alleviate some discomfort. But more than likely you will leave the office empty handed. As most doctors suggest doing the things I've listed and they won't break out the prescription pad unless there is a medical need. Apparently mom being uncomfortable is not a medical emergency.

HEMORRHOIDS

Completing the list of conditions that start with H is the all too dreaded hemorrhoids. Not only are these uncomfortable and make bowel movements painful, they are also embarrassing when you are getting romantic (ahhem) with your husband.

So what are they? Why do they show up? Your body is struggling to accommodate the extra blood volume that you have when you are pregnant. If you haven't noticed any stressed out veins on the skin's surface (perhaps an increase in spider veins or varicose veins), it doesn't mean that they aren't there. Everything that is located in your body that shuffles blood through it (aka your circulatory system) is enlarging to make way for the extra blood volume.

Complicating matters is your growing uterus. As your uterus grows, it places additional pressure on the pelvic veins, especially the inferior vena cava, which is a large vein on the right side of the body that receives the blood from the lower limbs (why doctors suggest pregnant women sleep on their left side).

And of course there's the fact that you are probably more constipated than usual thanks to your super slow digestive tract. Constipation can cause or at the very least, complicate hemorrhoids. Straining while trying to have a bowel movement can lead to the development of hemorrhoids as you place added stress on the veins located there.

But there is help for the hemorrhoids!

1. First and most important...you must try to avoid constipation as much as possible. HAHAHAHAHAH. Sorry I had to laugh here. Constipation is really hard to avoid. But you can eat a high-fiber diet which will help move your bowels (slowly) through the digestive tract, drink water which helps keep your bowel hydrated to help ease it through, and get regular doctor-approved exercise. If you are really bothered by constipation, ask your doctor he/she may be able to give you something to help uhh EASE the pain ☺.
2. Don't keep a bowel movement in. When you feel the urge, rush to the bathroom.
3. Don't push or strain while having a bowel movement.
4. Do your daily Kegel exercises. These are helpful because they increase circulation to the rectal area and strengthen the muscles there.
5. Avoid sitting or standing for long periods of time. If you are on bed rest, elevate the legs and increase the blood flow to your lower extremities.

What if you've done everything you can, and the hemorrhoids still come? There are things you can do to relieve the pain and discomfort. Here are some pointers…

1. Apply ice. Ahhhh frozen butt. Yes, I know it probably doesn't sound fun but ice is great at reducing swelling and discomfort. Wrap ice with a soft covering to avoid direct contact with the skin and apply it 15 minutes on, 90 minutes off.
2. Soak in the tub. Soak in your bathtub for 10 to 15 minutes a few times each day. If you don't have a tub you can purchase a sitz bath at the store.
3. Gently and thoroughly clean the backside area after each bowel movement. The best thing to use to clean this delicate area is a soft, unscented white toilet tissue. Don't

use colored or scented varieties because these can cause irritation.
4. Moisten the tissue if needed.
5. And of course, as your doctor or healthcare provider to recommend a safe topical anesthetic or medicated suppository to help relieve discomfort. Don't buy one without his/her approval. Even medications applied to the skin are absorbed into the body, bloodstream, and eventually babies.
6. Relax. These annoying little buggers will go away after delivery. Not right after but over time they will get smaller and eventually disappear. If they don't, your doctor can recommend stronger medications once the babies are born and/or possible surgery.

Now that we've learned about the three H symptoms, it's time to discuss the three L symptoms. Because great things come in threes!

LOVELY LEG CRAMPS

Beginning our list of L symptoms is the lovely leg cramp. No one's really sure why leg cramps are common during pregnancy, but your additional pregnancy weight and pressure from your growing uterus could be to blame. These leg cramps could come at any hour of the day. These leg cramps are more noticeable at night but are present throughout the day. And as your belly grows, these cramps can get worse. So what can you to about them?
Prevent them.
   •   Try to avoid sitting or standing with your legs crossed. Pay attention to your feet and make sure you keep them shoulder width apart at all times for optimum circulation.
   •   Give your calf muscles a nice stretch regularly during the day and several times before you go to bed. Simply put one foot in front of the other like you are going to

do a lunge and lean forward grabbing onto something for support. Press your lean through the hip area but try to avoid bending at the hip. Keep your back foot firmly planted on the ground behind you and you will feel the stretch in that calf muscle as you press your weight forward through the front hip area. Or if you'd rather sit, put your feet on an ottoman or other surface in front of you and dorsiflex the foot, pulling the toes in toward you while pressing the heel away from you.

- Keep your ankles in motion by rotating them and wiggle your toes when you sit for any period of time.
- Take a walk every day, unless you are on bed rest or have been advised not to.
- Lie down on your left side.
- Drink plenty of water to stay hydrated

When the cramp comes...

If the cramp comes anyways, there are some things you can do to help relieve the pain. First, you must immediately and carefully stretch your calf muscle. The best stretch after the pain comes is to straighten your leg and gently flex your foot by pulling the toes back towards your shins. There may be pain at first but the pain will gradually go away as the stretch works on the tight muscle that is experiencing a spasm.

If the stretch doesn't work, you can apply a nice and firm pressure to the area and massage the area. You can also try to apply heat to the area but be careful to avoid too much heat and only apply it for a short period of time-a few minutes. Walking or moving around may be helpful but it never helped me at all. Moving always made the cramp worse.

When to call the doctor.

Leg cramps can be a symptom of something more dangerous happening inside. A blood clot may have formed. If your pain is constant and not occasional, or if you see swelling and redness, or feel tenderness, or if the area is warm to the touch it is time to call the doctor. Although blood clots are rare, they are more common in pregnancies with multiples. And it's always better to be safe than sorry.

LOW BACK PAIN

Low back pain is all too common in pregnancy. When you are pregnant with multiples, it seems a lot worse than when you are pregnant with a singleton pregnancy. Low back pain can be more apparent at times when the babies press against your spine. Other times it might be barely noticeable at all. The pain may stay in your back or may move to your pelvis and butt area.

Hormones loosen all the joints and ligaments that attach the hip to the spine. This makes you feel out of balance and this loosened tissue causes great discomfort when you walk, sit, stand, lift, or switch positions. Yes, in other words, these ligaments and joints cause pain pretty much all day long.

There are two patterns of low back pain during pregnancy; Lumbar pain and posterior pelvic pain. Lumbar pain is felt in the lower back at the lumbar spine and posterior pelvic pain is felt in the back of the pelvis. Both are quite painful and both should go away within a few months of the birth.

First, don't make the pain worse. If you are experiencing pain over and around your lower spine, you have lumbar pain. To avoid making the symptoms worse, do not sit or stand for long periods of time. Also, avoid lifting anything heavy. Lumber pain sometimes radiates down the leg.

If you are experiencing pain lower than your lumbar spine, deep inside the butt area or on one or both sides of the back of your thighs, you have posterior pelvic pain. To avoid making symptoms worse, stay away from activities like climbing stairs, walking, getting in and out of a chair, switching sides you are laying on in bed, and twisting. Also avoid positions where you bend at the waist, particularly leaning forward while working at a desk.

Often people who experience back pain think it's a condition called sciatica. However, true sciatica only affects about 1% of pregnant women. Sciatica isn't just lower back pain, it's pain that radiates down the leg and makes the leg pain worse than the back pain. It also can cause pain to your foot and toes and create numbness. If this is the case, consult your physician and call him/her immediately if you lose sensation or you experience weakness in one or both legs, or lose feeling in your bladder, groin, or anus.

What to do about back pain.

1. Avoid activities that make it worse. Listen to your body and avoid aggravating your back pain.
2. Exercise. Although you may want to crawl in bed and spend the majority of your day there, exercise is precisely what you need to alleviate the back pain. Unless you have been put on bed rest, movement is just what the doctors order to help back pain. Strengthening exercises will help build the muscles that surround and support the spine, stretching exercises will help keep the supporting muscles flexible, and walking will help keep your body warm and active and help you feel less stress. So get moving and get that back pain outta there!
3. Do pelvic tilts. Get on your hands and knees with your arms shoulder-width apart and your knees about hip-width apart. Now, keeping your elbows straight but

not locked, tuck your buttocks under and at the same time round your back as you breathe in. Then relax your back and allow it to return to a neutral position as you breathe out. Repeat in a slow and controlled manner.

Exercise safely. Here is a checklist of safety tips to help you exercise safely while pregnant…

1 Check with your doctor first
2 Make sure you take in adequate calories.
3 Avoid dangerous sports where there is an increased risk of falling or injury. Don't bike outdoors. Use a stationary bike. Don't do any contact sports or sports where an object is thrown in your direction. Never roller blade or skateboard, and don't go swimming in the choppy ocean waters.
4 Warm up and cool down before and after every exercise session.
5 Stay hydrated by drinking a minimum of 8 oz. of water every 10-15 minutes while exercising.
6 Listen to your body and don't overdo it. If at any time you feel like you are having trouble breathing, you feel lightheaded, or you experience pain…stop.
7 Don't ever lie flat on your back.
8 Get up from the floor slowly.
9 Avoid exercising in the heat.

Be aware of proper positioning and body mechanics throughout the day.

1. Stand up straight and hold your body in proper postural alignment. This gets more challenging as your body changes but always try to keep your pelvis slightly titled in and your shoulders back. Avoid the temptation to slump your shoulders and arch your back as this puts more strain and pressure on the spine.

2. Don't sit for extended periods of time and don't stand for extended periods of time. Keep moving throughout the day.
3. Wear comfortable footwear. Avoid high heels.
4. Always use proper lifting techniques by bending at the knees while lifting things to minimize the stress on your back. Don't reach for items too high. Ask for help.
5. Keep balanced. If you are carrying grocery bags, evenly distribute the weight between both sides of your body.
6. Be careful getting in and out of bed. I had to develop a roll to accomplish this task. I bent my legs and rolled out of bed. I used my arms to assist by pushing myself up as I dangled my lower legs off the side of the bed. It was fun...
7. Sleep on your side with your knees bent and a pillow tucked between your thighs.

ROUND LIGAMENT PAIN

Finalizing the list of L symptoms, and completing the list of most common pains during pregnancy, is round ligament pain. This pain can show up as a quick, sharp, and stabbing pain or it can present as a longer lasting dull ache. This pain is felt in the lower abdomen and groin area and begins in the second trimester with a singleton pregnancy. However, with a multiple pregnancy it can begin late in the first trimester.

What are they? The round ligaments surround your uterus. As your uterus expands during pregnancy, the round ligaments get stretched and thicken to accommodate and support your uterus.

As these ligaments change, they may cause pain or discomfort on one or both sides of your uterus. These pains are noticeable with getting out of a chair or your bed or when you roll over to switch sides in bed. You may also feel them while getting out of a chair or getting out of the bathtub. Also if you have had a hectic day you may feel them as a dull ache as you are winding down.

Unfortunately because this pain is located in the uterus, you must call your doctor if you experience four episodes or more of this pain within an hour. It could signal that labor has begun.

Also, another common labor sign that can mimic round ligament pain is low back pain. If you are experiencing low back pain or pressure in the pelvic area you should contact your doctor.

Round ligament pain by itself is not an alarm for anything. It is temporary, comes and goes, and will stop shortly after the babies are born. However because it is pain located in and around the uterus, round ligament pain has a danger that it can hide true labor pains. So if you are ever in doubt, just call your doctor. It is always better to be safe than sorry.

You can get some relief from round ligament pain. First, when pain strikes, sit down or lie down and take a break. Try to relax. You can also try to flex your knees toward your abdomen to help stretch the ligaments or lie on your side with a pillow underneath your uterus and another pillow between your legs. Listen to your body and find what method works for you.

HORMONES FROM H**L

If you could pinpoint one culprit that begins the process of all h**l breaking loose within your body while pregnant, it would be HORMONES. Pregnancy causes a mega chemical imbalance within the body. You are working so hard at nurturing another life inside of you that it causes hormones within you to go haywire as your body works double time to care for your developing infant. Compounding matters is when you are pregnant with multiples as this imbalance can get to be downright disastrous. You now attempt to live a "normal" life as a totally abnormal person. But sit down, relax, and breathe. This craziness is only temporary and although it gets rough at times don't check yourself into the insane asylum just yet. Believe it or not, there are things you can do to help balance those raging hormones out and level off your chemicals to a somewhat manageable state.

So… what exactly are hormones? Hormones are the body's chemical messaging system. Hormones transport information throughout the body in the blood, organs, and tissues and affect numerous body functions. Some of the processes altered by hormones include

1. Mood stabilization
2. Procreation
3. Sexual desire
4. Metabolism (the breakdown of food for use as energy)
5. Physical development and growth

Hormones are created in the endocrine glands. These include the pancreas, adrenal glands, thyroid, thymus, pineal, pituitary, and testes and ovaries. The endocrine glands make up the endocrine system. It's like the endocrine system is its own separate interstate of special cells within the body. These glands work together and the slightest alteration in the amount of hormone content running through your body can have a huge impact on several body functions.

After you conceived your twin wonders, the balance of hormones changes and can trigger many systems to go haywire. These hormones include:

1. Human Chorionic Gonadotropin (hCG)-Aahh the wonderful hormone that the pregnancy test detected to make the second line appear on the test stick. Typically the production of this hormone starts 11 days after conception. It's the hormone that begins all the trouble within your endocrine system. hCG is the hormone responsible for the cessation of your monthly menstrual cycle. And it leads to increased production of two other hormones-progesterone and estrogen. Did you notice your moodiness accelerated toward the end of your first trimester? That's because production of this hormone is highest between your 8th and 11th week. But fear not, this hormone does level off and decrease in intensity into the second and third trimester...unless you have twins. Double baby means double hormones!

2. Progesterone-The hormone hCG began the trouble but watch out for the hormone Progesterone that is next in line on your way to the loony bin. This hormone is responsible for a safe and successful pregnancy. Progesterone creates the environment for healthy egg fertilization and helps the womb support the egg properly. Your boobs get bigger due to this hormone as progesterone triggers milk production.

3. Estrogen-You may have always heard that estrogen is the hormone responsible for all our female problems. But as you can read above, estrogen is only one hormone in line of a list of several hormones that cause us trouble. Estrogen helps support the fetus by increasing thickness of the lining of the womb to protect the growing baby. Estrogen causes blood production to increase so that adequate blood can travel to the breasts and womb. And estrogen is responsible for all the awesome muscles that relax and get flexible so that your body can make way for your growing uterus. Unfortunately estrogen causes some of those aches and pains that you experience as your womb expands because those muscles, ligaments, and tendons will stretch to new lengths and create an environment for injury and pain. So always move with caution because literally you have a brand new body that you are moving around in.

4. Oxytocin-This hormone will not be elevated until just before delivery. Oxytocin triggers the contractions that begin labor. It helps after delivery to shrink the womb back to its original pre-pregnancy size. Oxytocin also aids in nursing as it causes a contraction in the breasts that allows the milk to be squeezed out by your suckling infant.

5. Relaxin-The placenta produces a hormone called relaxin that does exactly what its names for-relaxes. Your body needs to get loose to accommodate your growing uterus. Relaxin relaxes the intrauterine ligaments and allows expanding of the uterus and pelvis during pregnancy. Relaxin also relaxes other parts of the body including the arteries. The arteries have to relax to accommodate a much higher blood volume. If the hormone relaxin isn't present, your blood pressure would shoot through the roof. Relaxin supports the hemodynamic changes that occur during pregnancy, such as increased cardiac output and increased renal blood flow. Finally the fun

of relaxin is that it relaxes your digestive system that causes those wonderful nights and days of heartburn.

6. Human placental lactogen: This hormone, also referred to as HPL, is another hormonal helper that prepares your breasts for lactation regardless of whether you decide to nurse. HPL causes the secretion of colostrum, the protein and antibody-rich yellowish pre-milk stuff that your breasts make before true milk comes in. HPL also changes the maternal metabolism so a pregnant mom can use more fatty acids and less glucose so that these substances are readily available for the growing baby. When you are pregnant with twins, this hormone is what causes a higher risk of gestational diabetes. HPL works with estrogen and the hormone cortisol to block the action of insulin, elevating blood sugar levels, starting around 20 weeks of pregnancy. You will notice that with twins you get to be checked more often for gestational diabetes. This is because if the pancreas can't pump out enough insulin to compensate for the changes triggered by HPL you may get gestational diabetes. Also, if you have gestational diabetes, it can be a warning inside your body that the pancreas is not as efficient as it should be. When you have birthed your twin wonders, talk with your doctor to make lifestyle changes to prevent diabetes from returning in your future.

Sex
One of two things can happen to your sex life while you are pregnant with twins. It can either get better or get worse. Personally I experienced increased sexual desire throughout my twin pregnancy. My body felt like hell but I wanted to have more sex. Figure that one out…I couldn't. And my husband was scared to have sex with me. So we were instantly NOT on the same page. AT ALL. And the arguments commenced.

The only thing unique in a marriage is the sex. Sex is the one thing the two of you share that you do not share with anyone else. It is a covenant seal of marriage. Sex is what a husband and wife do to seal their marriage vows on their wedding night. You can talk and spend time doing the same things with your spouse that you can share with a friend or relative. Except the sex. This is why sex is a very important element of a healthy and happy marriage.

As you get further along, you will notice that positions during sex are quite a challenge. Being pregnant with twins can actually make your sex life fairly boring. Moving into several positions can get uncomfortable and you will find that the further along you get, the less positions you will be able to enjoy. But here's a news flash for you…it isn't about the multitude of positions you can cram your body into. It's about the emotional, physical, and spiritual connection the two of you share. I have put together another list ☺. Hopefully you will find some pointers to help keep that spark lit in your sex life.

1. Take it nice and slow. Sex is something that is enjoyable when it is slowed down. Take time with each other and learn to be gentle during sex so that you don't hurt each other. If you are going too fast slow down. Many sensations during sex are stronger when you take extra time to feel them. My husband can drive me crazy with just the slightest touch. He has brought me to orgasm on several occasions by being very gentle and slow. Give your marriage a chance to experience all the sensations you can feel during sex. Slow down.

2. Set the mood. Sex for a man can start at the point of the first turn on. Sex for a woman can start at the beginning of the day. What a couple does in the beginning of the day can have a direct impact on the bedroom mood at night. So setting the mood isn't just

about lighting candles and playing slow soft music. Setting the mood is an emotional process that begins at the start of your day. Begin the day by taking a few minutes with each other to say "good morning." Kiss for extra time than you normally spend kissing. Hug a little bit longer. Send sexy text messages back and forth when you are separated through the day. Get off the computer, Facebook, and turn off the television. Cut out distractions especially as nighttime approaches. Men have the ability to make or break the day. So men...it's pretty much in your hands for this one. Don't come home from work with a bad attitude. Don't get right into fixing the items on your to do list. Just come home, get showered and changed, and invest some time in your wife. Wives, this is not time for mopping and spring-cleaning. Get everything done before your husband arrives at home. And if you are at work, follow the advice I gave to the husbands.

3. Get your stomach in order. The worst thing for sex is a grumbling and unsettled stomach. Especially when your husband is on top, gas gets triggered quickly. There is so much added pressure on your intestines that if you are using the man on top position gas is triggered because of the added pressure from his weight. It's embarrassing. By now you should know what triggers your stomach to be upset (umm..everything). Eat carefully throughout the day, avoid gassy foods, drink plenty of water, and avoid processed foods. When I was pregnant with the twins salad was a big gas trigger. I had to opt for steamed green beans or sometimes skip the veggies entirely if I wanted to have a special night with my husband. It is worth skipping vegetables and your favorite foods to have sex with each other. What good are vegetables going to do for you if your marriage is in shambles from not spending time together? Everything has to get in balance. That means sometimes stepping back and looking at the BIG picture.

4. Experiment with positions. Toward the end of pregnancy I had only two positions I could be placed in to enjoy sex. The first position was a great one as I was able to have an orgasm. The second position was mainly for my husband's enjoyment. Because I hated it. We tried several positions during my pregnancy. But as the weeks went by so did the possibility of different positions. I was limited by my belly. And he was limited because he was always afraid he was hurting me.

    a. The best position during the pregnancy for me and for most other pregnant couples out there is the woman on top position. On top, you can control the depth of penetration and maneuver your husband to touch the areas that feel good to you. If you take time and experiment with positions and depth of penetration you will find out how to bring each other pleasures and have a great orgasm together. I know, this is a really private thing to write about in a book, but I feel like you should have the right information. Sex between a husband and wife is a powerful thing that the two of you share. Without it, your relationship can get rocky rather quickly. There may be a point where you have to quit having sex. So enjoy it while you are allowed to partake. It strengthens your bond.

    b. The other position we could use while I was pregnant was the position where he was entering me from behind. I would lay my stomach on the bed as I was draped over, or lay on the bed flat. As I got really big I had to get on all fours. This is a terrible position for me. I hate it. I feel degraded in this position. But my husband really enjoys it. For many husbands this is their favorite position. So we used this position on the days I knew I wasn't feeling the best anyways. In other words, on days we both knew I might not have an orgasm because life's worries were crowding in my head.

Remember you are to have sex for your husband and he is to have sex for you. There is nothing wrong with getting into HIS favorite position ☺.

5. Play. As you get bigger, sex becomes more challenging. Embrace the challenge. Shop around and find some sexy outfits and/or toys to use while having sex. I personally purchased 3 new baby dolls (these fit the best with an expanding belly) while I was pregnant. When I put them on they made me feel better. I was able to relax more because I felt more attractive to my husband. He liked them too. Especially as he took them off of me. He also learned what to wear to help me get in the mood. Confidence is probably the most difficult mountain you will need to climb while having sex together. You will feel less confident as you get a larger belly. So have fun and buy some sexy stuff to wear. And if you're really brave find some fun toys to use. Sex was given to a husband and wife for their pleasure. If you have to use other items for now, don't worry. Your normal sex life will return shortly after you've recovered from childbirth. And who knows? Maybe these items will remain a fun part of your love life.

6. Enjoy. And of course the most important part-enjoy. Enjoy each other during this time. Some people are very turned on by pregnant women. Most husbands agree that a pregnant woman who is carrying their child is one of the sexiest things they have ever encountered. So wives, enjoy your husbands. Husbands, enjoy your wives. Do what makes you both feel good. Aim to have that quality sex life you've always dreamed of having. It is literally all in your attitude and approach. So keep your chin up, smile, and enjoy, enjoy. enjoy.

Immobility

I seriously thought I wanted to go on bed rest…until I was put on it. My life was slightly chaotic so I figured being forced to say "no" to all the work ahead would be a breath of fresh air. I was wrong. IT WAS TERRIBLE. But with a twin pregnancy bed rest is virtually inevitable. So the best thing you can do is prepare to be lazy. And try to get some enjoyment during your upcoming R & R…

CHAPTER TWO
Surviving Bed Rest
When the doctor tells you it's time to rest.

Bed rest will save the life of your babies. Doctors argue back and forth over whether bed rest is necessary. Some say it doesn't prevent pre-term labor. Others say it does. Personally, bed rest saved my twins. And as awful as it was to be on it, I'm thankful my doctors insisted that I slow down and take extra time to rest.

There are three stages of bed rest. The goal is to follow the instructions of the first stage of bed rest-called modified bed rest. That way your doctor may not put you on the second or third stages. And the doctors are smart. They have been highly trained to have ESP and know whether you are following instructions or not. Well, not really, but they can tell by what your body is doing if you are resting or running. So don't try to get away with activity if you've been told to lay low. Your doctor may just skip stage two and put you right in the hospital for stage three-bed rest if he feels he needs to keep you in check. His/her goal is to deliver those babies healthy even if it means making momma miserable.

Modified bed rest is the first stage of bed rest-I call it bed rest stage one. Modified bed rest has some freedoms attached. You can drive the car, go to the bathroom, run small errands, and probably perform light housework. I was on modified bed rest for almost 20 weeks. It was a struggle for me because at the time I still boxed at the gym and lifted weights, I was in my final semester of my Exercise and Sports Science degree which required working at sports events, I volunteered as a basketball and soccer coach for middle school kids, and I held my own teen ministry in my home on Friday nights.

Additionally I had four boys at home. Their ages were 16, 11, 9, and 5. I was BUSY BUSY BUSY. And I did not have time in my daily schedule for rest. Well, guess what? I had to MAKE time. And that's what you might need to do too.

Surviving Modified Bed Rest

First, you should stockpile movies, books, and other items to prepare for possible upcoming bed rest. Bed rest is more likely after 16-20 weeks gestation so you should have some time to prepare. If you haven't begun already, gather a collection of items to help you survive lying around in bed. Snacks, magazines, crafts to busy your hands…keep them in a container and keep adding more. I added lotions and nail polishes in mine. Well, not really, I never did this…but if I had done the stockpile I would've added those items and made my life SO much easier.

Second, change your approach to being placed on bed rest. I thought I could catch up on my writing. But because I failed to prepare for bed rest I was not in the right mind-set to write. I literally wasted months of precious down time because I had a bad attitude. Prepare yourself mentally for bed rest and it will help you a lot for the "bed battle" ahead!

Before my twin pregnancy I had so much energy I could run circles around my children. No one could keep me from my daily bouts of intense bike rides, runs, and weight training sessions. My addiction was movement. Outside, inside, rain or shine…I was at peace while I was in motion. So to take several months and live a motionless life was the most awful thing I'd ever attempted to do. My mind couldn't handle the thought of rest, especially the thought of 5 or 6 months of it.

But the mind needed to change. My thinking was stinking. I approached bed rest like it was a death sentence. And resented every waking moment I was forced to be immobile. Sometimes I would get up out of rebellion and try to do something active. But my body would quickly remind me why I needed rest and I would reluctantly surrender back to my recliner or bed. It was a nightmare.

It is critical to survival that you have a positive approach to bed rest. It is estimated that over 700,000 pregnant women a year are put on bed rest (Maloni). And out of these 700,000 women a significant number suffer from some sort of antepartum (before baby is born) and postpartum (after baby is born) depression as a result of their bed rest. As far as I can tell, no one has died on bed rest of boredom or insanity…at least I couldn't find any statistic on this. So keeping the right attitude can make the difference between feeling like you are a queen at the top of a castle and feeling like a prisoner in the bottom of a dark dungeon.

The goal of modified bed rest is to prevent going to the next phase, stage two, which is bed-rest with bathroom privileges…yikes. Modified bed rest means you need to rest when possible, however you will not be confined to a bed. You will have to cut out the running around, modify your shopping habits, and recruit help for the house. Normally you can still have sex with your husband and have normal showering/bathroom privileges. With a little ingenuity modified bed rest can work for you.

Home on modified bed rest.

You should find a comfortable recliner, or purchase one if you don't have anywhere comfy to sit. You will be doing lots of sitting. The recliner is a great investment because it will also serve a purpose once your twins arrive. It also helps your circulation as it provides an area where you can put your feet up. When you aren't on your comfy chair you should be in your bed. Those are the places you can 'rest'. Get used to them, set stations up for water, snacks, and items to grab to keep you busy. And enjoy. Let life happen around you and only get up when it's necessary.

Out and about on modified bed rest.

When you go anywhere you must choose to sit. That means if it's at a friend's house, plop on his/her couch, at the doctor's office stay seated in the waiting room, and if you go to church travel straight in and sit down. Socializing will need to be kept to a minimum. I am a social bug. So for me this was very difficult to do. It seemed many people who were used to my level of chit chatting also had trouble adjusting to my new quiet and reserved lifestyle. Some are still offended to this day, assuming I am angry with them just because I stopped chatting with them.

Shopping on modified bed rest.

This is when I had the most fun. Shopping. Why? The electric wheelchair, of course. Choose to shop where there is an available electric wheelchair for you to use. When you get to the store, get in it and go! Shopping on foot can trigger pre-term labor. The added stress of being in the store, especially if you have other kids with you, can be overwhelming for your body. Resting your body in the wheelchair while your mind is going 100 miles an hour with all the buying decisions can literally save your little babies' lives.

I learned to enjoy the wheelchairs at the stores so much I had my favorite ones picked out. I shopped most often at the grocery store where the wheelchair was the fastest. My second favorite store had the wheelchair that could maneuver around everything with precision. I tried to make it as fun as I could. I would get close to the other shoppers but not too close that I would hit them. I turned the corners like I was in a racecar. I even sometimes made engine-revving noises. I wanted to make it look like it was fun so that I could enjoy the time I had in the chair. And it did look life fun because my kids wanted to ride in one too! Which of course became an argument ☺.

Modified bed rest is an opportunity. An opportunity for you to get caught up on life things that you may have had no time for previously and prepare you for the upcoming birth. It is also a great test, a test to see how the rest of the family is going to handle extra work for them. Twins does not mean double work for MOM…no, it means extra work for EVERYONE…

Recruit help for your modified bed rest.

Recruit help for the house. It is time for a system my friend. You need to develop a system that works for you and your family to help keep the house tidy and get the chores done. Since you are immobile, this is a great test run for what is to come. And enjoy it while it lasts. I'm back 100% now and I fight to keep my kids and husband helping with the housework. I find the more chores I do today, the less they do. It's in their nature. So tighten up ship and make lists, lists, and more lists.

Before my twins were born, I lived in a household FULL of boys. And they were lazy boys. When I was placed on modified bed rest I had to delegate jobs. Before the bed rest I did almost everything in the house. It was my fault my family was lazy. I had decided long ago that if I wanted things in my house done right, I would have to do them myself. And I did do it myself. So when it came time for the family to pitch in, they were virtually clueless on what to do. Looking back on it, I see how they really do like to and want to help. And although it is still a struggle, they've all become much better at pitching in and lightening the load on me. I seriously couldn't do the TWIN thing without them!

Here is a sample list of who did what in my home. You can certainly use it to tidy up your own home or create your own list. First, you write down everything that needs to be done for the household on a daily, as needed, and weekly basis. Then you delegate jobs. Try to pick the person who would be best for the job, not necessarily the oldest ones. Oh…and you might want to call it the "job" or "duty" list, not chore chart. Kids get hives when you mention the word "chore".

If you don't have other children, you and your husband need to sit down and go through the duties of the house item by item and come up with a game plan. This plan will be implemented until at least 3 months after your babies are born while you are recovering from the pregnancy and birth. So make it a plan that works for BOTH of you.

- ✓ Consider lawn service. We live in a townhouse. My husband doesn't have a yard to take care of so it's easier for him to work inside the house and help me with the chores. If you aren't fortunate to have lawn service, you may want to consider hiring someone. If money is tight, hire a neighborhood kid to come around once a week and trim the grass. You will be surprised at how much more your husband will do inside the house once you've relieved him of the lawn care duties outside. Remember, this is about survival. And drastic times call for drastic measures. Keep the lawn service after the babies are born so he can continue to help you.

✓ Get a laundry system in place that works for you. My husband washed and dried the clothes in the washer and dryer and then placed the clean clothes next to me so I could fold and hang them. He still does this today. He does the physically demanding part (moving the loads) and I do the part that's important to me-keeping wrinkles out of the clothes. It works for us. Try it; it might work for you too.

✓ Dinner is done! Keep dinner simple. Now that you're limited you will not be able to fix five-course meals. Ha-ha, I never did anyways. But I'm sure you get what I'm saying here. Hang up the apron lady (what's an apron?), It's time to make dinner simple simple simple.

✓ Grill. My husband loves to grill. We ate a lot of grilled chicken, fish, and steak while I was pregnant. You will want to support him by making side dishes a breeze. But with a little preparation, dinner can get done. Find out what type of cooking your husband loves and encourage him by complimenting his food dishes, even if they don't taste very good.

✓ Purchase easy foods. I had to retire the Spanish rice pot and bought boil in bag rice or single serving yellow rice with easy to follow instructions to cook instead. We bought lots of frozen French fries and potato dishes instead of peeling our own fresh. We bought canned or frozen vegetables instead of fresh. We bought ready-made salad kits instead of fresh items separately. And we saved money to spend on take-out food when necessary.

✓ Make dinner clean up easy. We had to simplify meal clean up. We opted to purchase lots of paper dishes and made sure we had an abundance of dishwasher soap.

But there will be times when you must help with dinner. If you do help, place a chair in front of the counter and do everything from a seated position. Always think "sit, sit, and sit." That's what modified bed rest is…sitting. As you get further along you will probably have to rest a lot anyways so you might as well get used to it now while you still have your sanity ☺.

Vacuuming and Mopping can get done, too. My husband bought a better vacuum while I was pregnant so that he or the kids could vacuum. They vacuumed upstairs and downstairs, tile and carpet. No one else mopped like I did so honestly I would mop from a chair. I'm kind of nuts about my tile floors and I have a special non-residue cleaner I use on it. But I did buy a nicer mop so it wouldn't be so hard on my body when I used it.

Cleaning surfaces and bathrooms. For this, I put paper towels and cleaner in each bathroom, and kept a bottle of cleaner handy by the tables downstairs. I bought extra spray bottles, filled them, and labeled them. Then I trained the family to pitch in and use it. However, I ended up doing a lot of the cleaning in the bathrooms while I was at the sink brushing my teeth or using the shower or toilet. It took me an extra minute or two as long as I kept up with it. My youngest son did the dusting downstairs. I used the same cleaner as I used on the floor for my surfaces. Shaklee's H2 cleaner. It works well for the family and it is harmless to the babies. You might as well prepare now for a cleaner house so purchase a safe cleaner to use for all your cleaning jobs. Have your husband, father, or hired help replace moldy caulking wherever possible. And inspect the house for any water damage that might have a potential to grow mildew.

This is NOT the time for spring cleaning or organizing. Just let go of it. Allow your family to do this for you, hire a cleaner, or let it go until you are released from bed rest. Either way it will eventually get done. So don't worry. It's TEMPORARY!

The second stage of bed rest is stage two-bed rest with bathroom privileges. This can be worse than stage three because in stage three you are in the hospital completely oblivious to the neglected condition of your home. In stage two bed rest you are fully aware of what is happening in your 'absence'. It is enough to make anyone crazy. Hopefully you've developed a great system on modified bed rest because now it's time to give your to-do list to someone else.

And that's about all you can do...give everything to someone else to do. You can't even do light housework from your bed. You are only allowed up for bathroom and possible shower privileges. Rest is rest. Period.

Also during this stage chances are you won't be allowed to have sex. This is a great challenge for a marriage because a man's greatest need is the need to have sex. And you are his wife whom he expects to do this with. Complicating matters, you are hormonal and probably a little bit paranoid that he might find it with someone else. Even the most faithful men are human. I recommend going through a marriage program on the television or purchasing some marriage counseling d.v.d.s or c.d.s and in place of sex take advantage of some learning time in the comfort of your own home. Use this as an opportunity to grow your marriage in other areas. Also, if he really needs to have sex, there are ways he can be satisfied without increasing the risk to the babies. This is a time to get creative with your husband. And remember it is worth sacrificing everything to have those babies come out healthy. You will be back to normal activity sooner than you think! Further in this book is a great section on saving your marriage through this time. Read it before the babies come. Marriage is a constant sacrifice of give and take. And it takes work. Together you can make it!

The third stage of bed rest is stage three-hospital bed rest. And for wisdom on this, I turn to my cousin who was on hospital bed rest for months before delivering her boy-girl twins. Jodi…what advice do you have to give here?

Jodi was on hospital bed rest for 7 weeks. She is also a nurse in the Neonatal Intensive Care Unit. She is probably more qualified than most people to give advice on stage three bed rest…here's what she had to say about her experience…

"Being a NICU nurse had its pros and cons while on bed-rest. I was dilated to 1cm. at 24 Weeks and taken off work. I knew what difficulties a 24-week baby faced, let alone two of them. Weeks in the hospital, questionable survival, and potential life long problems (head bleeds, CP, NEC, ROP). I told Mike, "I CAN'T have 24 week twins". I was admitted to the hospital at 28 Weeks, and delivered at 34Weeks 6 days. I was dilated to 6cm. for the last two weeks. Because I had seen first hand what a difference a day makes for an unborn child, I followed my doctor's orders exactly. **I can't tell you how many babies were born too soon because mom convinced her doctor to let her get up to shower against his better judgment and then she went into labor**. I showered twice a week, and those were the fastest showers of my life. One very experienced highly thought of obstetrician said it was amazing that I was dilated to 6cm. with twins and was still going strong. My point is to **STAY IN THAT BED!!!!** As hard as it may be on the mom for another week, day, or even minute, it is more difficult on that baby for a LIFETIME if it is born too soon. A day does matter! Every day matters to that fetus. If I hadn't listened, if I hadn't been a NICU nurse and knew the importance of every day I could give them, my babies' lives would be vastly different than they are now. They are healthy! And that is worth any amount of bedrest, greasy hair and smelly pits!"

Jodi did have her challenges in the hospital. She has another child and it was very difficult to arrange visits with her. For any hospital stay, the worst part is being away from the children. Jodi visited with her other child only once a week!

"I tried to put a positive spin on things and that helped get me through it, like I finally had things in life I'd always wanted...a maid (housekeeping) cleaned my room daily, I had a personal chef (not gourmet, mind you, but a chef nonetheless), and I lived in a gated community (hospital security). Mike picked up my laundry and brought it back, so I had a laundry service, and I never once in 7 Weeks had to do dishes. I caught up on all the chick flicks I wanted to see. A great woman that worked with me brought movies in for me that I picked out from a list she gave me of movies she owned. I took a nap everyday. Sounds great when you look at it that way, but the absolute worst part was being away from my daughter Ellie. I'm tearing up now just thinking about it 6 years later. She was shuffled around from Mikes nieces (Michelle) house to my sister's house weekly while Mike was at work. Mike worked evenings, so he'd drop Ellie off at Michelle's Monday through Wednesday at 2 and pick her up at 10. On Thursdays he took her to my sister's house at 2, she'd spend the night there so he could grocery shop Friday morning and then work and he'd pick her back up Saturday morning. Because he was so busy at home and running her everywhere, he could only bring her to see me once a week. That was really hard. She was exposed to shingles and wasn't allowed to visit me for 3 weeks because of the risk of infecting someone else on the unit (chickenpox and shingles are the same virus and are both very dangerous to unborn fetuses if the mom has never had chicken pox). I hated that! I cried for Ellie daily (never told anybody that). I missed her so much and felt horrible that her world was turned upside down and she had to deal with it without her mommy. She had nightmares every night until the day I came home. The first night I was home in my bed was the first night her and Mike had slept uninterrupted for 7 weeks (babies were still hospitalized). Since I was hospitalized in the same place I worked, she would tell people I was at work, and when I went back to work after delivering she asked me daily for 6 months if I was coming back home :(she thought I was going to be gone for weeks again. I also remember telling Mike to tell her that I was the sick one not to blame it on the babies, I didn't want her to hold it against them. She was 3 1/2 at the time. One of my NICU coworkers brought cinnamon ice cream in for me and kept it in the freezer on our unit, so when Ellie came one Saturday, I called the NICU and had them bring us some. They brought it in a plastic mug and to this day every time someone uses it, Ellie will say, "that's the cup I ate ice cream with mommy from when she was in the hospital". I will never throw that cup away."

So what is the bottom line advice for bed rest? No matter what stage you are in you must approach it with a positive attitude, follow it exactly as you have been told to, and use it to your advantage to recruit the extra help you need once the twins are born. Enjoy bed rest, take advantage of the down time, and adhere to your doctor's instructions. You have only one pregnancy with these twins to get through. Make sure it's worth every moment by carrying those babies as long as you can!

CHAPTER THREE
Getting ready for the big day
What items you really need for two (besides a third arm).

Saving Energy
The travel system

My husband and I searched high and low for a travel system that would be practical for our family. This travel system needed to have two bases, two car seats, and a double stroller. Because we were on a budget, we had to piece our system together. Although there are some twin systems available, as soon as an item says "twin" it triples in price. I'd advise for you to get creative and put together items for singletons and make them work for two. Your mind and your pocket will feel so much better about the price.

But the travel system is a must-have for twins. This system allows you to take the baby seat out of the base that is secured in the car and place the seat in the stroller. This can be done without disturbing your sleeping or content baby. If you can't afford one ask for help in getting one. The car seats we purchased were $110.00 each. But they were worth it for us. And we put the stroller that the seats fit into on our baby registry. That way it broke up the cost for us. Your basic travel system brand new and pieced together (because they don't come ready made for twins) is about $370.00. That includes the double stroller, two car seats, and seat bases for the car.

The travel system is a lifesaver in so many ways. I come home from dropping the kids off at school and I put the babies right from the car into the stroller. Then we hit the local fitness trail for a brisk walk.

Sometimes those walks are the only peace I have in my day. And as the babies got older they became much more aware of their surroundings and enjoyed the fresh air.

When I go to the grocery store by myself with the twins (yes, I can do that and so can you), I usually bring the stroller inside the store with me. I've gotten very good at balancing a hand-held grocery basket on the stroller. When I have help at the store I recruit one of my kids to push the stroller or the cart. Now they argue over who gets to push the stroller, they enjoy it so much. And we get the shopping done in record time. If I have a lot of shopping to do and I have brought along help, we put the car seats in two grocery carts. Sometimes it's so easy that the babies sleep through the whole store. They love their car seats. We attract a lot of attention in the store but twins always do. So allow for extra time! Oh, and bring emergency bottles just in case ☺.

Saving Space

Consider space savers and purchase only what you need for the stage your baby is in.

Stuff, stuff, and more stuff. There's a ton of stuff that babies require throughout their infancy and into toddler-hood. Swings, bouncer seats, exercisers, mats, high chairs, carriers, and tons of toys to grab. But relax, take a deep breath, and stop worrying. All the items aren't needed at once. And with twins, buying products in age stages will save you space AND money.

New babies don't need stuff. They need clothes, blankets, and diapers. With twins you will need a place to put them in because you don't have a third arm. But I have some sensible tips on just what to do to help you keep your pocketbook full and your sanity intact.

Crib and Playpen. You need to purchase a crib and playpen with diapering in mind. Newborn babies require about 10-12 diaper changes per 24-hour period. With twins that number doubles. Your greatest challenge besides feeding will be keeping up with the diaper changes. A majority of your diaper changes will be done as the babies wake up. And having them sleep near diapering areas is a big help to get you through.

Purchase a crib with a changing table attached. Purchase a crib with a changing table attached. Purchase a crib with a changing table attached. Purchase a crib with a changing table attached. GOT IT???

There are two areas you will need a place to lay your sleepy babies down. The first area is the nursery. My twins still sleep in the same crib. In the hospital the nurses put them in the same crib. The twins will sleep better, at least until they are moving around, if they are put in the same bed together. We purchased a great looking crib with changing table attached for $200.00. They aren't much more expensive than regular cribs. At first you won't need two cribs so take the extra cash and buy diapers. YOU WILL NEED THEM.

The crib also has extra shelves behind the changing table and a roll out hamper. We absolutely swear by it. We just leave one in the crib while we diaper the other and then we switch them. Easy easy easy. Really, it is.

The second area is the living room. This is where you will need a Pac 'n' play type playpen. Get the one that has a bassinet and changing table. The bassinet is a part of the Pac 'n' play playpen that makes an additional high surface for the babies to lie on. This is crucial so you don't have to bend forward far to get to them. And the changing table part just flips over the side when not in use. Mine even has a diaper stacker and baby wipe area. It cost us around $80.00 and I LOVE IT.

Swing and Bouncer. You will need a swing and/or bouncer seat for each newborn. Although they are too young to bounce or swing, it's a great place to set down a baby as you tend to another, and you will want these items portable. We purchased a bouncer seat/space saving swing in one. This was also a lifesaver. It was around $55.00. The only downfall was that when I was recovering from my c-section I had a difficult time getting the babies in and out because the space saver we bought was low to the ground. But all in all we were happy with the decision. It has saved us a lot of aggravation and space.

Bathtub. We purchased a great bathtub with a sling inside of it that can be removed. Another lifesaver. Really. You won't need two tubs because you won't be bathing two at the same time, especially in the beginning. We started out bathing our beauties in the nursery on the floor. We placed towels down on the floor and put the tub on the top of the towels. It was just easier to do it on the floor. At first you won't be able to submerge the babies because of the umbilical cord area. After that falls off you will be free to fill the tub up. But always watch the babies and do not take your eyes off of them while they are near water. Ever.

Accessories. A small collection of accessories will go a long way. Here is a list of necessary items and then a list of "should haves"...

Necessary-
    Baby Bath and shampoo
    Baby powder
    Diapers diapers and more diapers (3 boxes minimum of
newborn)
    Two boxes of 100 count or higher baby wipes
    Two wipes containers (one for crib one for bassinet)
    Infant ibuprofen just in case one gets ill and doctor
    suggests using it (it will also be helpful for those first
    shots). But anytime your newborn has a fever you
    must call your doctor and not play dr. mom at home.

    Bottle of Electrolyte Replacement
    Cotton Balls
    Rubbing alcohol (For the umbilical area if it gets wet or
    looks red)_
    Bottles (even if you are breast feeding you will want to
    have these on hand)
    Slow flow nipples for bottles
    Formula in case you need to supplement your milk or
    have chosen to formula feed
    Diaper bag or two with portable diaper changing pad
    (get one for dad also…he probably doesn't want a girly
    one though)
    Baby nail clippers
    Baby brush

Should haves-
    Diaper rash ointment (so far I haven't used this)
    Bandages for babies
    Pacifiers (at first I used these it helped calm them down
    but now they've both found their thumbs)
    Baby monitor for nursery
    Head roll protectors for car seats

All the items listed above are the items you will need for the first several months. As your babies grow you will need to add more items to your collection. I know this may seem overwhelming but it really isn't. Twins just make you get more organized, something I struggled with for almost 40 years until I had them. And this brings us right to the next section, which I hope you can utilize…saving money.

Saving money

Shop closeouts online and consignment shops. Tell visitors to bring diapers and baby wipes

Are you eligible for WIC? Medical insurance assistance? You are going to need all the financial help you can get. Because I quit working after I was placed on bed rest, my husband and I qualified for the WIC program and additional assistance. The WIC program is a government program that provides formula, baby foods, cereals, and food for mom. When breastfeeding failed for me at 6 weeks postpartum, I had to put the babies on formula. WIC provided me with 10 cans of formula per baby each month. At $16.00/can that saved us $320.00 every month. Plus the other foods like milk, eggs, cheese, cereals, and vegetables helped shave off $50.00 from our $700.00/month food bill for the family. The WIC program was a lifesaver in our household.

Are you eligible for Medicaid? Search the Internet for the state run Medicaid program in your area and apply. Florida groups food stamps with Medicaid so we were able to apply for both at the same time. We didn't need help with these programs with both of us working. But once the twins came we desperately scrounged around just to feed our kids. Often my husband and I wouldn't eat just to put food on the table for them.

When I applied I got full medical for my kids (saved us about $200.00 a month to leave them off my husband's medical insurance), and $430.00 in food assistance. So sucking up my pride and applying for help saved our household a total of **$1010.00** every month. **That's over a thousand dollars every month.** And our temporary situation is what these programs were designed for. Today we don't use these programs any more as we can afford to pay for items with cash. But I urge you, if you are eligible for some help, use it for a temporary time. Your tax dollars have been pouring into these programs to help other people. Don't pass by an opportunity to use it for yourself.

Find shoppers and set them out to shop for you. My husband's sister Dawn and his mother Ricki LOVE to shop. I can't stand to shop. I prefer to Internet shop or not shop at all. I get hives when I enter the mall. But my sister-in-law and mother-in-law absolutely love to spend countless hours shopping for the best deals. So when the twin girls were born, they set out weekly to shop the sales and consignment shops to provide us with wonderful items for our babies. It is one of our greatest blessings!

Shopping for twins can be fun if you love to shop. But dragging them out with you can sometimes be a nightmare. You may find that it is difficult to concentrate on shopping because people will constantly interrupt you to admire the babies. If you are lucky and able to hide behind the clothing racks where no one can spot the twins, then chances are one baby will protest being out.

And of course, there's the germ risk. Strangers ALWAYS grab the babies' hands and the babies ALWAYS stick those hands in their mouths. UGH!!! GERMS!!!! So, if possible, leave those bundles of joy at home or let someone else do the shopping for you.

Consignment shops are a great resource if you don't mind used baby items. This is best when they are really little because most newborns barely wear their clothes and often items get resold brand new. Whatever items you purchase, make sure you bring those items home and wash them in baby detergent. Consignment shops don't have washers and dryers and will put items on the shelves as is.

Consignment shops are also great places to shop as the twins get older. When they grow out of items times TWO it is wonderful to turn those items into a consignment shop and either take cash or trade them in for the next thing you need. Consignment shops will deal with your used items by either giving you cash on the spot, allowing you to trade in for other items, or giving you a percentage of the revenue your used items bring in. Shop around for the consignment shop that will deal with you and your items in a way that works for you.

Saving sanity

Having twins does not mean double work for mom it means extra work for EVERYONE.

If possible, you will need to store up vacation time for the arrival of the twins. By now you may have figured it out that there will be no two-working parent household with twins on the way. If you haven't been put on bed rest by now, chances are you will be. For us bed rest was a great practice run for what we would encounter ahead. It's about saving your sanity now, not about taking the greatest family vacations. There will be plenty of chances to do that in the future when the twins are older.

So how do you save your sanity? Just a little planning ahead and you will be well on your way to total twin success!

First, you need to take a survey of how many people are potential helpers in your household. This begins with the children. If you have other children, it's time to recruit their help. I recommend paying them a small allowance to help out with the household chores that would normally be done by mom or dad. Kids want to help. But there is a fine balance between keeping them interested in helping, and making them resent you for every little chore you bark out. Kids are all different and all will react differently to chores. When the twins arrive there won't be extra time at all for you to do many of the daily items the household requires to be maintained.

1. Pick out chores the kids do not do very well or chores you have to do. For us, the kids can do everything except scrub toilets, mop the tile floors, and clean the kitchen. We decided to do these chores because I want them done right. And although my kids can probably clean those areas too, it also makes them happy they don't have to do everything in the house.
2. Decide on what the kids can and can't do with the babies. My kids can do everything with the babies except change their diapers and give them a bath. They often argue over whose turn it is to give the babies their bottles.
3. Reward them for pitching in. The reality is...kids will want to help if they are given some type of compensation for their help. I know what you're thinking and I know many of the child experts will roll their eyes at this. Why do we need to reward our kids for working? Well, think about it this way. If you went to a job and worked for 8 hours, would you work for free? If you didn't get rewarded in the form of a paycheck, would it make you want to quit working? And how would your quality of work be if you had to work for free? Kids need to get rewarded. It's teaching them to expect a certain level of reward for their work in the future. Remember, you aren't raising kids, you are creating adults ☺. Reward

them...it will make your life SO MUCH easier. And they deserve it!

2 floor solutions for two

This section is for those readers who live in a multi-level home. One of the greatest challenges you will face when you are recovering from twin childbirth is conquering the staircase. So your objective will be to make that trip upstairs less often. It will save you time and energy. And to do this, you must come up with an effective game plan for 2 floors!

And I have the flu to thank for this section...really. When I was in the hospital recovering from my c-section, two of my kids tested positive for influenza type H1N1. They had high fevers (102-103.5) so I sent my husband to the E.R. four floors down from the O.B. ward while I stayed in my room. I suspected it was the flu but I wanted to be sure. Well, sure I was. They tested positive for flu, were given some prescriptions for medicine that was about $1000.00 and were sent home to rest. We couldn't believe how sick they were. It was a nightmare. My twins' pediatrician suggested I find somewhere else to go when I was released from the hospital. But instead we opted to isolate the floor upstairs to flu. And the two-floor system for the twins worked so well we are still using it today.

Babies have three biggest needs on a daily basis. These are sleeping, eating, and pooping/urinating. With these three things in mind you can create two floors that work for you and minimize that climb up and down the stairs. This is very helpful because when you bring those twins home you will be absolutely exhausted. Plus climbing those stairs can be a challenge when you are recovering from a c-section.

✓ First, set up a sleeping and diaper changing area downstairs. Hopefully you have one set up upstairs. Ours on the second floor was the crib/changing table that we bought and swear by as a lifesaver. However, downstairs we had to come up with another solution. We have a small house and 8 people living in it. So we had to save space and utilize a system that would work for us.

Enter the Pac 'n' play. Ours had a changing table and diaper stacker attached. Bingo! It was a blessing and to this day we still use it a lot. There is NO WAY that I am climbing my stairs just to change diapers. NO WAY. We only use the upstairs changing table before we lay the twins down for bed and before we take them downstairs in the morning. Other than that, we use the Pac 'n' play changing table and couldn't imagine life without it...seriously.

✓ Second, add an area where you can store diapers, baby, wipes, baby blankets, and extra baby clothes downstairs. We have a ½ bath downstairs and have extra room in it. So we bought a little shelving system that rolls to put the extra diapers, wipes, and outfits in. It is canvas and cost around $12.00. If you don't have room for something extra, make room under a sink or in the kitchen to store stuff. Our Pac 'n' Play stores about a day's worth of diapers and a whole container of wipes. So if you can't arrange space anywhere else, just bring down enough stuff for the day from upstairs every morning. And if all else fails, use the bottom part of the playpen for diapers and wipes storage. It's not the prettiest solution but it works!

✓ Third, bring down a hamper. You will need it! When my twins were new, we switched their outfits at least 2 times every day. Plus with visitors coming in and out, we felt it necessary to switch out blankets and clothes every time they left. I know it probably didn't do much for germ control but I am a germ freak so it worked for me. A hamper or basket is small enough to place under an end table or sofa table. And it will eliminate many of those trips up and down. You should already have set up an area for extra clothes and blankets. So pitch the old dirty stuff in the hamper and break out the new ones. You can do all this without climbing up one step!

✓ Fourth, set up a comfy rocking chair. I spend a lot of time in the rocking chair downstairs. When the twins were first born the chair was in the nursery for overnight feedings. However, once they began sleeping through the night, there was no need to keep the chair upstairs. So I moved it down. And I used it AT LEAST 6 times a day...everyday. Now my twins LOVE to rock. I position each twin facing away from me on each hip. Their legs straddle my legs so they each get a firm grip-one straddles the right leg the other straddles my left leg. And then once I've assured they are secure, the rocking begins. Usually they are out and sleeping soundly within five minutes of rocking.

✓ Fifth, get a feeding plan. Whether you are nursing, supplementing, or both...you will need to set up a feeding plan to utilize quickly and efficiently on both levels of your home. Since we don't have an upstairs kitchen and I hung up the nursing 6 weeks after the twins were born, we had to make an area upstairs to help us with the feedings. We had water, formula, bottle liners, and clean nipples ready to go. Now at four months old, the twins only eat downstairs. But for a few months it got hectic to keep up with their frequent feedings.

In the beginning, it is difficult to figure out how many bottles will be needed overnight. If you are supplementing, you will need to place formula, water, and bottles upstairs to assist you with the midnight wake ups. What you should do is set up one of those small 3 drawer plastic containers that you can purchase for around $13.00 in the room. Then, put bottles pre-measured with water in one drawer, keep plastic bags for dirty diapers in another drawer, and keep the third drawer empty for dirty bottles. As an added bonus, I suggest putting some ready to feed bottles in as well with some nipples. If you are exhausted you will not want to mix formula at 3 a.m. so putting some ready to feed bottles in your feeding supply is a big help. In the morning, just grab the dirty bottles from the third drawer and take them downstairs with you to clean. And at night, bring more pre-filled bottles, liners, water, and formula upstairs with you to replenish the supply.

✓ And lastly...bring the baby swings downstairs. Downstairs is where we keep most of our extra baby furniture. The swings are downstairs and now the exersaucers are downstairs. Since we only go upstairs to bed, there is no need for these items to remain on the 2nd floor unless I need extra space downstairs for visitors. I tuck them away in a far unused corner of my dining room when these items aren't in use. The twins love people. So even today they'd rather be held then placed in the exersaucer or swing. But I still take time out every day to place them in these items. I need the break and I also want them to stop being so dependant on me to hold them. So far it's working really well. I've returned to normal chores around the house and I even get time in my day to work on my writing.

So, with a little creativity and planning, you can survive twins with a multi floor home. Commit to climbing those stairs only when necessary and it will not only save energy, it will also help you recover faster from childbirth. Always plan to bring things you will need downstairs with you when you go down. And bring the stuff you will need upstairs when you go up. I even set up a stair dedicated to things that needed to go upstairs so that when I went up, I'd just scoop up my little collection. And I did the same thing upstairs as well. I like my new system and I still use it today ☺.

Section two-The Babies Arrive

CHAPTER FOUR
The day the World Changed
The Arrival of my Twins.

Surviving Childbirth for two

My girls, Brooke and Esther, were born via c-section delivery on May 30, 2012 at 8:30a.m. and at 8:32a.m. It literally was the day my world changed.

I had never had a c-section before. I watched several videos to find out what to expect but nothing prepared me for what could go wrong. And things DID go wrong.

We had to be at the hospital for my planned c-section at 5 a.m. So of course I didn't sleep all night. I was anxious for my babies to be born so that I could breathe and feel better and I was afraid I would oversleep and miss the alarm. I tossed and turned until I got up to take a shower at 4 a.m. It was time to go.

We had done several tests the day before at the hospital. They had drawn my blood, taken my vitals, height and weight, and I sat down with the anesthesiologists. I am a faithful person, relying on prayer and God to help me get through scary situations. But to be quite honest, I was absolutely terrified. The thing that scared me the most was the spinal. The doctors were going to place a long needle in my back and deliver the anesthesia that would block the pain of the surgery. I know enough about the body to understand that there were some risks involved.

But I had no choice in the matter. C-section was the safest way to have the babies. And since my last child got injured to his brachial plexus during delivery and suffered a paralyzed arm, and I suffered a back injury, I knew it was the best option for me. Even though I was terrified.

When we arrived at the hospital, we were quickly brought to our room. That room would be the room I was going to spend the next four days in. They hooked me up to the monitors one more time to check heart rates and contractions, and then prepped me for surgery. Surgery prep involved the following steps…

1. I.V. They hooked my arm up to an I.V. This I.V. would stay in place until the 3rd day. It was used "just in case" they needed to deliver drugs to me in an emergency. Also, it was an easier way for them to deliver pain medications.
2. Bicitra. This is an acid neutralizer they gave me before surgery to help prevent any vomiting. Although I hadn't eaten for the last 12 hours there was a chance that I would still vomit during the procedure. Well I did. It was fun because I didn't have anything to vomit. So dry heaves while they are cutting open your midsection to pull babies out is definitely not a picnic in the park.
3. Consult. You will have your consult with the anesthesiologist and he/she will go over explaining the procedure once again. Most planned c-sections require a spinal tap. However an epidural can be used if the c-section isn't planned or in some other cases where the doctor requests it. Both numb you from the rib cage down. And both require an injection of the medicine into your spine. Don't worry though. You will be numbed first. They will usually do the injection in the operating room.
4. Husband suits up. It's time for the work for hubby. Before you make the trip to the operating room, they will have your husband or significant other suit up for

surgery. He will put on scrubs including a gown, cap, and shoe covers. He will make the trip down the hall with you so you won't be alone.

And now you are ready to go. Most of the big stuff happens in the operating room. So they will wheel you on a bed down to the O.R. where you will have another series of steps.

1. They will place you on the operating table. This was a weird experience for me because I was so big and the table was so small. I guess comfort was not on the surgeon team's mind when they chose the table to operate on. But for me this was the first thing I noticed. I felt like I was going to fall off

2. Surgery team prepares you for surgery. Your doctors will come in at the last minute. So several nurses and assistants will prepare you for the surgery. You should have at least one or two anesthesiologists, about 2 or 3 nurses for you, a nurse and/or pediatrician for each baby, a surgery assistant that will be in charge of the scalpels and scissors for the procedure, and your support. In other words, you will have a small army in your operating room before the doctor even shows up.

3. There will be lots of action in the room. I had two obstetricians attending my surgery so of course there was a discussion about where they were. When the nurses confirmed the doctors had arrived at the hospital, they finished prepping me for the surgery.

4. They will put you draped over your knees on the side of the operating table while they deliver your spinal. They will numb the area (mine was numbed by a small injection) and then deliver the drugs. DO NOT MOVE. This is the most important time to be still. Once they are finished administering the anesthesia, they will lay you down on the table because you are numb from the rib cage down and won't be able to do it yourself.

5. Catheter. Now the team of nurses will insert your catheter. No worries here because you can't feel it. The

catheter will stay in place for about 24 hours after surgery until the feeling returns in your lower body. My catheter was placed wrong and I have trouble to this day with sensitivity down there. I couldn't have any control over it though because I was at the mercy of the nurses placing it.

6. Drape. They will place a drape between your face and the surgery area so you cannot see. This was probably a pretty freaky part for me. I had no idea what was happening because I couldn't feel anything or see anything.

7. Support. You should have your support person at your head during the procedure to help hold your hand. My husband was unable to be in the room but the anesthesiologist positioned herself at my shoulders and held me so I wouldn't be scared. The entire time during the surgery she kept checking to see if I could feel certain areas on my chest and shoulders by placing stickers and then taking them off. She wanted to make sure the numbing drugs weren't working TOO well. Apparently sometimes the spinal will travel more towards the head and make the doctors freak out and hook you up to a machine that will help you breathe. Fortunately all was good with this part.

8. The surgery. I had 6 natural childbirths before embarking into the c-section world. So I was fairly nervous during the actual procedure. It seemed like it took forever and there wasn't pain but I could feel some pulling for the first few minutes. I had heard horror stories about c-sections gone bad. I found myself wishing that they could give me more drugs and knock me out completely. Being wide-awake and having no idea what people are doing to your body is a pretty scary experience.

So what is going on under that curtain? And why all the commotion??

Here are the normal steps the doctors take for a c-section. If you are pregnant with twins you will probably not have an emergency c-section. The doctors have already figured out if you are a candidate by the position of the babies and if you can deliver them naturally. So relax and let the doctors do their work.

1. More prepping. They will either shave your pubic area in the room or on the operating table. They will also disinfect the area so that the doctors will have a sanitary surface to work with. Surgery can introduce all types of infections into the body. Having a clean and well-groomed incision site is crucial to keeping the bad stuff out and the good stuff in.

2. Incision. Under normal circumstances, the incision should be about a middle finger in length. My incision is almost twice as big. But it doesn't bother me because I really can't see it. They knew my babies were fairly large so they cut me a little wider to get at the babies safely. Also I was getting my tubes tied so they needed to see in there ☺. Don't worry so much about the incision site. Twin skin takes some time to get rid of and your scar will fade before you know it!

3. The incision does not go through the muscle. The surgeon cuts away layers of skin and fascia, and then makes the cut into the uterus. Your abdominal muscles go the sides while you are pregnant towards the end of your pregnancy. They stretch sometimes up to 8cm. and then they separate. I used to tease people and say I do crunches but my whole body goes sideways. This actually isn't far from the truth. Just like when you go through a curtain in the center and the panels move to the sides as you push past, the same happens with your abdominal muscles as your uterus grows and pushes past. They stretch to the sides. So when you are cut for c-section the abdominal muscles are not cut they are simply moved to

the sides if they are in the way. Making after baby abdominal exercise no different recovering from a c-section than from a natural birth.

4. Reaching baby A. By now you've heard baby A-baby B for quite some time. This refers to which baby comes out first. The doctor will locate the head of baby A, cuff his/her hand around it, and push on the top of the uterus to push the head down and out. You might feel some tugging here but shouldn't feel pain. This is when I started to puke. The nurse had a pan nearby so she turned my head and the small bit of saliva came out. As quickly as nausea came on it disappeared.

5. Baby A will cry. The doctor will clamp and cut the cord and hand the baby over to the nurses. The nurses will work on the first baby. I still hadn't seen Esther-my baby A. They waited until her sister got out to show me both babies together.

6. Baby B will come out next. The doctors will repeat the same procedure. Once the nurses clean up both babies they will bring them over to you. This was the crappiest part of c-section. I couldn't go skin to skin with the babies. I was still technically "in surgery" so they had to keep me clear of others, including my babies, as they continued to work on me. So I got a drive-by glance at Esther and Brooke before they wheeled them into my room.

7. Now the fun begins. Both are out, both are safe. But now they have to get out the one or two placentas, perform any other cutting if you are getting a tubal, and stitch you back up. You will probably feel tugging here but before you know if they will wheel you out of the O.R. and bring you to those beautiful twins you've waited so long to see.

If you are still feeling squeamish after you've read the description about the surgery, I am going to suggest a few methods I wish I'd have used to help me prepare for my c-section. I believe that education is key to getting rid of fears. The unknowns are always scary. But once you teach yourself about what to expect you will find your fears will virtually go away. Educate yourself educate yourself educate yourself.

1. Watch c-section surgeries on a video viewing platform on the Internet like YouTube. Pick the ones that are less graphic and less bloody. Even animated ones might help you.

2. Search for an interactive c-section video and do the surgery yourself. The more educated and familiar you are with the c-section the less afraid you will be on your big day. I like the virtual c-section video at http://www.surgerysquad.com/surgeries/virtual-c-section-cesarean-surgery/

   I wish I had discovered this great tool before I got my surgery. This website actually allows you to interact with the animated patient and perform the surgery again and again. Making you a c-section expert by the time delivery day comes around.

Not all twins are born via c-section. Whether or not you will have a c-section largely depends on the position of your babies in the last trimester. My twin A was using my cervix as a bouncy seat, in a position called "frank breech". There was no way I was going to deliver vaginally. Twin A (Esther) didn't want to stop looking at her sister. To this day, Esther loves to look at her sister's face. This apparently was the case while they were inside of me because she simply wouldn't budge from her difficult to deliver position. Twin B (Brooke) was in a beautiful head down position ready for exit. Unfortunately if twin A is uncooperative, there is no way they will deliver the twins vaginally. For me it was the best option because after all is over and my recovery has been complete, I feel no different than I would've after a regular vaginal delivery except I'm definitely not as flat tummied as I used to be.

Will you have a c-section? Chances are you will. If you have twins in the same amniotic sac you will. If they are in separate sacks, your chances are still in favor of having them by c-section. Now, I've read several articles of the possibilities of getting a c-section while you are pregnant with twins and they basically tell you that having twins doesn't require c-section. However, what they don't tell you is the fact that some doctors insist when there are twins to not attempt a vaginal delivery. Period. No matter what position the babies are in. Personally I'm glad we delivered via c-section. My babies came out perfectly healthy and not injured at all. Although I had some minor complications it was nice to avoid squeezing two heads out and avoid labor. Labor for twins is longer and harder. Sorry to lay down the truth here but I'm not sugar coating anything for you. C-section is a great option. Don't be afraid of it if your doctor wants to deliver the twins that way. And most doctors will deliver twins by c-section at your request.

The facts are that although 40% of twins are positioned in a head down-head down presentation that is ideal for vaginal delivery, there has been a dramatic increase in the rate of c-section deliveries for twins. The rate was at 53% back just 12 years ago but has shot up with new estimates as high as 75%! This is because the injury risk to twins is much less when delivering via c-section. Even in the most ideal position for vaginal delivery twins can change position while in labor and can cause things to go terribly wrong.

There are risks involved with any surgery and c-section does carry many of those risks. They include risk of infection, risk of damage to the bowel or bladder, and increased risk of respiratory problems with the infant. However with twins it is just as risky in certain cases to have them vaginally.

With my experience in delivering naturally and delivering via c-section, I do not think the c-section was any worse than regular delivery. My body did take longer to heal from the c-section but only because I suffered with Pregnancy Induced Hypertension and was placed back in the hospital to get that under control. But my PIH was with me in the last trimester so it wasn't anything brought on by the c-section. Once I had the babies they could deliver better blood pressure reducing drugs to me. And it took 6 weeks postpartum to be weaned off the blood pressure drugs. So if I look back and take my PIH out of the scenario, my c-section was easier than vaginal delivery. Yes, that's right…EASIER than vaginal delivery.

The ideal position of the twins, the position you probably look for sonogram after sonogram, is the head down-head down. Baby A and Baby B will more likely be delivered vaginally if both babies are in a head down position. If your doctor will not deliver them vaginally and insists on taking them out via c-section, listen to him/her. Don't go off on a rant about banning the c-section. There is nothing you will be able to do to change his/her mind.

And even if twin A is delivered vaginally, there is a chance that twin B could flip after twin A is birthed. Your doctor has his/her experience and reasons so do not go against the doctor's advice. Your doctor has done this before and knows why a c-section is best.

Any other positioning of the twins warrants a c-section. If twin A is head down and twin B is breech, there is a chance that you will have both a vaginal and c-section delivery. It happened to one of my obstetricians. She pushed out twin A but twin B wouldn't turn around and head for the exit. Her recovery was terrible because she was recovering from two kinds of birth.

If twin A is breech and twin B is head down, there is an increased risk of both heads getting stuck in the birth canal together. It has happened more times than you think it does. Don't risk this dangerous birth. Insist on a c-section here. When both heads enter the birth canal together, they will usually need to sacrifice one or both babies just to save you. This is the worst scenario and don't think it can't happen. I strongly recommend doing a c-section in this case. If your doctor refuses (which shouldn't happen with twins), get a second opinion. This is the one case where I suggest arguing with your doctor.

If twin A is breech and twin B is breech at 35 weeks it is time to discuss c-section with your doctor. It's highly unlikely that both will turn because if you hadn't noticed already-you are running out of room. The twins don't have much space inside to be able to do a complete 180. It is time for the argument of "are these babies done cooking yet?" An argument I will help you with in the section below.

My doctor and I had the discussion for weeks. He wasn't willing to get the twins out until 39 weeks. I was in mild labor from 36 weeks on. But it didn't matter. My doctor did not want to budge on the date for delivery. He felt that the best chance my babies would have is if they stayed inside for as long as possible. Even though I was dying on the inside. This was a difficult time for me. I was in so much pain, I hadn't slept well for over a month, and I had some difficulty breathing. My twin A was "frank breech" which means she was sitting with her backside on the bottom of the uterus. Her butt was literally plugging my cervix. My cervix was thinning but was nice and closed. My twins were comfortable inside, even though I was not.

I tried to talk to the other doctors about going in for c-section before 39 weeks. They wouldn't budge either. I was so frustrated that I wanted to change doctors. I had read several articles and all of them stated full term for twins was between 36 and 37 weeks gestation. No one put 39 weeks! UGH!

At 36 weeks I got some hope for an earlier delivery. I WAS IN LABOR!! ☺ I downloaded a contraction monitor for my phone (I recommend this) and timed my contractions. In the morning the contractions would start 20 minutes apart and last 45 seconds. Then they would get closer together in a definite sequence. 15 minutes apart, 10 minutes apart. By mid-afternoon I was timing painful 5-minute apart contractions that lasted 90 seconds. I knew it was real labor. I even passed my mucous plug. Now I was very happy. Time to go in and have these babies. OR SO I THOUGHT…

Some women can't progress into full labor with a frank breech baby. I didn't know this until the twins. The doctors wouldn't even see me. My cervix only opened 2 cm. in two weeks of labor. My contractions would be 5 minutes apart, and then they would spread back out again until they were 20 minutes apart. And the next day, the same thing would happen. Over and over again for 2 weeks. For labor to open a closed and healthy cervix, the baby's head or feet need to be positioned at the cervix and as the uterus contracts it pulls the baby's head or feet down and that pressure dilates the cervix. My baby A was still using my cervix as a hammock in a frank breech position so there was nothing being pushed down into the cervix to stimulate dilation.

With twins you must be so careful to let your doctors know right away if you feel you are in labor. They will generally know the position of the babies and will also know if it is time to bring you to the hospital. Call right away if your contractions are getting closer together or if you have a bloody show or gush of water. If you can't get in touch with the doctor, call again. Read about the warning signs of labor, and if you are still in doubt, just go in and be seen. It is always better to be safe than sorry.

Did you know that your body actually prepares for labor about 4 weeks before labor begins? There are several signs that indicate your body is preparing, but these signs do not necessarily warrant a call to the doctor. Just monitor and take note of these events and call your doctor when in doubt.

1. You note more Braxton Hick contractions. These might get closer together just like mine did. However, if they do not get longer, stronger, and closer together along with dilating the cervix they are not true labor contractions. Just keep track of them like I did and call the doctor if these contractions are accompanied by a gush of water, a steady trickling of water, or bleeding.

2. Your baby drops. Not literally, but you will notice increased pressure in the bottom of your pelvis, and you may notice in the mirror that your belly has all of a sudden gotten lower. This means baby A is dropping into a position for birth. And it also means that those Braxton Hicks contractions will soon progress into real labor. This is a normal event and does not warrant a call to the doctor.

3. Your cervix begins to dilate. Some women can walk around with a dilated cervix for weeks but when you are carrying twins the doctors will probably admit you to the hospital if your cervix dilates beyond 2 cm. It is normal for your cervix to dilate up to 2 cm. before real labor actually begins, especially if you've had babies before. In the last month leading up to delivery your doctor may do a vaginal exam or two, just to check your cervix to see if it is dilating beyond 2cm.

4. Passing of the mucous plug. This is definitely a good sign that labor is near. Your mucous plug is a thick substance that lies at your cervix to add an extra layer of protection for your babies. It has literally plugged your cervix during the first 8 months of your pregnancy. As the cervix thins and begins to open, the plug gets released and will come out. Some women notice an increase of vaginal discharge some notice discharge tinted with blood, and others notice it coming out in one nice yucky clump. Mine came out in one nice yucky clump. It wasn't colored at all. It just looked like a big blob of Vaseline. YUCK. You don't need to call the doctor on this unless bleeding accompanies your plug. Not just tinted mucous but blood. My doctor didn't care that I passed my plug. I felt like saving it for my next visit and throwing it in his face.

5. Your water breaks. I used to believe that my water would break in one big gush and I'd soak everything around me in a matter of seconds. This has never ever happened to me. Unless your cervix is dilated open, your water will not gush out. It is more of a trickle or steady light flow.

And it is so confusing. When you are in your last trimester of pregnancy you notice it is much more difficult to control your bladder. Often a cough or sneeze will be enough of a movement to cause a trickle of urine. When your water breaks it often mimics this same light urine trickle. The way to tell if it is really your water leaking is if this trickle does not stop no matter what you do. If you lay down, it still trickles. You have to use the bathroom every few minutes because it still trickles. If your trickle doesn't stop it is time to call the doctor. If you are in doubt, it is time to call the doctor. But even in the hospital it is difficult to tell if it is amniotic fluid or urine. They test the fluid but sometimes it doesn't show up as amniotic fluid. With my fourth child I knew it was my water but the test showed no fluid. I sat in that hospital and insisted they retest. They did and they found amniotic fluid. You are your advocate. Make sure if people are not "getting it" that you speak up and demand they take care of you properly.

Labor contractions can come and go but if there is a steady climb towards longer and closer together pains, then chances are you're in labor. The general rule of thumb for a normal singleton pregnancy is to call the doctor or go into the birthing location when your contractions last about a minute each and come every five minutes for an hour. However, because you are carrying twins, you might be instructed to come in earlier, like when they are 7 minutes apart. You will have to talk to your doctor and find out when he/she wants you to call. Every situation is unique. Do not ever sit home and disobey doctor's orders. And of course if you are in doubt, go in and get checked. It is always best to be safe than sorry.

CHAPTER FIVE
The Aftermath
Surviving the hospital stay

What I felt after. This was a pretty scary time for me because I didn't know what to expect. The biggest fear I had was the fear of not getting the feeling back in my legs. It took me almost 24 hours for the feeling to return. The nurses would poke me in different areas and see if I could feel the pokes but I did not. They regularly checked my legs. I was getting more afraid. They didn't think it was a big deal that I had no feeling in my lower body. I was terrified. But after I went to sleep overnight the first night I woke to feeling some of those pokes. And as the day progressed I felt more and more pokes until I could finally get up and walk.

They put my babies in my hospital room and had them under the warmer waiting for me to arrive. My husband was with the babies while they were still sewing me closed in the operating room. I had such a terrible time with my pregnancy and since I'd had eight kids, I felt that it was time to tie those tubes. So my surgery took about 20 extra minutes as they were completing my tubal.

When they wheeled me in my hospital room I was still fairly groggy from the morphine they give you during and after the c-section. I was also really confused. I couldn't feel anything from the bottom of my ribcage down. And I knew I had a catheter in so that didn't add to any comfort. But I was relieved that the babies were out because for the first time in a long time…I could actually BREATHE!

I think when you are pregnant with twins it really doesn't hit you until you see your new babies. I looked over at my bundles for the first time and couldn't believe my eyes. They were so cute! And they looked JUST LIKE each other. They were big, too. Esther-twin A weighed in at 6 lbs. 14 oz. and Brooke-twin B weighed in at 6 lbs. They were in separate cribs under the warmer but that would be the only time they would be separated as we would soon realize they relied on being with each other for everything. They were quiet and taking in their new surroundings. The nurses shuffling around them were so happy. The entire staff at the hospital seemed to delight in the new twins. And so did I.

My husband was the happiest I'd ever seen him, except for the day we got married. He just kept staring at Esther and Brooke, and thought they were the most precious things he'd ever seen. He was crying he was so happy. And so was I. All this time I thought it would be so hard to have twins and take care of two babies. But from what I was witnessing I realized that twins were the most content babies I'd ever seen. And over the course of the next several months I would discover that having two wasn't any more difficult than one. What a gift from God, and what a special day for all of us.

The next several days would be spent in the hospital, entertaining visitors, getting regular check-ups, and spending time with the two new babies. But with the good stuff and all the wonderfulness that we experienced, there were some bad moments too. And now that I've been through it all, I'd like to share some of insight with you.

Preparation
I'm sure you've read articles with lists after lists of what you should bring to the hospital. I know I did. Those lists were LONG. I didn't want to bring so much stuff with me. So I've revised a SHORTER list for those of you who don't feel like going to the hospital toting a huge suitcase of stuff with you.

WHAT TO BRING (REALLY)

1. A nightgown. Yes yes yes. Those hospital gowns are uncomfortable and hard to maneuver in. Bring a nightgown, a nursing one if you are breastfeeding. Make sure it is comfy and you have lots of room to move. Now is not the time to be fashionable. Now is the time to be COMFORTABLE.

2. A robe. This is great to have with you, especially if you are bleeding a lot and prefer to use the hospital gown for a couple of days because you don't want to risk ruining yours. The robe covers up the opening in the back so it's a must have for that hospital gown. Also as you get up and walk around the hospital you may get cold. Bring a nice soft robe and have it close to your bedside so you can grab it quickly. I found the pinkest and softest robe ever for about $10.00. I use it around the house to this day.

3. A bra. Your boobs get big and heavy, especially when your milk comes in. Get a nice bra and keep them supported. I opted for a nursing "sleep bra". It was so comfortable.

4. Hair ties. You hair will be somewhat messy as you are lying around in bed. Grab a few hair ties to help contain your locks.

5. Make up. Bring make up because you will have lots of visitors. Also bring a mirror and place it in your kit so you can pretty up right from the comfort of your own bed.

6. Big comfy underwear. The underwear they give you in the hospital is yucky. It's like a big fishing net. I suggest shopping for some very large cotton briefs to wear post-surgery or post-birth. Make sure the elastic band will sit high enough so that it will not irritate your incision site just in case you have a c-section. These beautiful 'granny panties' will be your best friend for a few weeks. So buy plenty and make sure you like them enough to actually wear them.

7. Socks. Nice comfy socks. For added stability you might want to purchase a pair with grips on the bottom. You

will be walking around a lot after the feeling returns to your legs. Your feet might get cold.

8. Slippers. Easy to slip on slippers. Make sure you can get them on and off without bending over and using your hands to assist. Keep them handy bedside for those walks around the halls. And make sure they are flat so that you won't lose your balance.

9. Emergency food. Although the hospital has plenty of food available upon request, you might want to have some comfort food handy for those long days in the hospital. Grab enough for both you and hubby. Frequent trips for him down to the cafeteria can add up quickly and drain you of money you will need. Pack smart and pack enough for a few days. Drinks should be available on demand at the hospital so you shouldn't have to worry about packing those.

10. Information. Bring the following items with you to the hospital...

    a. Pediatrician's phone number. If he/she doesn't visit in the hospital, you will need to call the office and report the birth. My twins' pediatrician visited every day to check on them. The first day we both got the girls mixed up because the nurses put them in the wrong crib.

    b. Insurance phone number. You must call your health insurance or Medicaid carrier and report the birth. That way benefits can start being paid immediately. Make sure you stress the fact that TWO babies were born. My insurance to this day is refusing to pay on certain bills because it has grouped my twin A and twin B into one i.d. number.

    c. Baby book if you are keeping one. This will be a great time to fill in all those blanks!

    d. Social security numbers for both parents. Any other insurance information that will be helpful. And if you are on the government program called "healthy start" you should call your representative and report the birth.

11. Shampoo, conditioner, soap, and razor. Although the hospital can supply you with these, there's nothing that feels better than using your own. Keep these items in a small bag and place them in the shower in your room.

12. Hair stuff. If your hair looks good, you look good. Sometimes you will want pictures of your new babies and you will be in those pictures. So keep your hair dryer, curling iron, straightening iron, and hair accessories handy. You will want them just in case.

13. Cell phone and charger.

14. Cameras and chargers.

15. Laptop or tablet so you can use the hospital's Wi-Fi.

16. Clothes for you to go home in. I wore the same outfit home as I wore in because I literally wore it for two hours on birthing day. If you aren't going to wear the same clothes, bring a very comfy outfit to wear home. Make sure it looks good on you and it fits. There will be lots of attention on you when you are wheeled downstairs with two babies in tow.

17. Outfits for the babies. Make sure these outfits keep them warm. Probably you will have to get preemie outfits. Even at full term my twins were only 6lbs. 14oz, and 6lbs. Regular newborn clothes overwhelmed their small bodies.

WHAT THE HOSPITAL SHOULD GIVE YOU

1. Crib card with their footprint, birth length, birth weight, and head circumference.

2. Bulb Syringe times two

3. Baby Wipes. Ask for extras because you have two babies.

4. Diapers. I got 5 packs of newborn diapers from the hospital when I took the twins home. The nurses just kept loading me up. Take all that the hospital will give to you. You will need lots of diapers for the first

several months because frequent diaper changes means less frequent diaper rashes.

5. Any bracelets or anklets with their hospital information.
6. B.P. cuff or any other medical items they dispose of. Just keep gathering stuff there's lots of items you can collect for the baby book.
7. Formula if you are formula feeding. Breast pump attachments if you are nursing. And they will give you supplies for both if you are supplementing and nursing.
8. Blankets, booties, hats. Some hospitals have handmade baby items they donate to every new baby. Because you have twins you will get double!
9. Pads and extra netted underwear for you.
10. Squeeze peri bottle. This is for washing every time after using the bathroom. It helps keep infection away and is essential for your take-home collection.

So now that you've prepared for your hospital stay and know what to expect when you leave, you are ready to live the 3 to 4 days at the hospital. How much time you spend at the hospital will be determined by a number of things, but ultimately that time frame is in your doctor's hands. Discuss the length of stay he expects you to have ahead of time and prepare for two extra days just in case. On my last day things went terribly wrong. I ended up spending an extra night at the hospital and I wanted to go home SO BAD. It was terrible.

Natural childbirth usually nets you once less day and night in the hospital. C-section is major surgery and they will have you stay at least an extra day. I know that everyone you talk to will probably tell you to "take it easy, rest, relax, enjoy the vacation."

But the reality is that this is definitely no vacation. If you aren't seeing the sandy beaches and sunsets in your hospital stay and are as miserable as I was, don't worry. THIS IS PERFECTLY NORMAL. I hate the hospital. HATE IT HATE IT HATE IT. I had two babies at a birthing center and I didn't even stay at a hospital to have them I hate hospitals so much.

But you can make your stay livable. Just pack your hospital bag and plan ahead. Find out what channels on TV the hospital provides in your room and check out the upcoming show schedule. Grab lots of cell phone and camera items to keep yourself busy. Bring your laptop and catch up on social networking. You will be better off if you keep busy especially if you're anything like me and hate hospitals.

Once you've prepared items for your stay, it is time to think people. Yes, people. The twins will bring LOTS of attention once they arrive. Get used to it, mine are almost 2 years old now and they are STILL attention hogs. Every single nurse had to visit my room. Friends and family came out of the woodwork to visit us in the hospital. Even the doctors liked to marvel at the babies and linger a little longer after they were done checking me. There was so much foot traffic in and out of my room that it seriously hindered my breastfeeding. So you must recruit your husband, mother, or close friend or other relative to be in charge of PR while you are in the hospital so that you can relax and get to do your greatest job-recovery.

After the babies are born, I suggest only allowing siblings and close relatives into your room. The first 24 hours whether you deliver natural or via c-section are very difficult. You are recovering from major childbirth...times two. Moving around a lot at this stage is not recommended. If you have visitors you will be more likely to move around. So for the first 24 hours, keep a majority of the massive visiting crew out of your room.

What recovery for the first 24 hours looks like...

C-section recovery. For the first 24 hours you may feel groggy and slightly nauseated. The pain medication is still circulating through your bloodstream and you will definitely not feel like yourself for several hours. You won't feel pain from the incision just yet but you might feel a little pain in your lower back as the anesthesia wears off and the area they stuck the needle in recovers sensitivity. I felt like a truck hit me as the anesthesia wore off but I couldn't feel much in my lower body until almost 24 hours later. I anxiously awaited the feeling to return to my legs and secretly wondered if it ever would.

The nurses will be in your room a lot for the first 24 hours. They will periodically check your vitals (blood pressure, temperature, respiratory rate) and they will press on your abdomen to ensure there are no places of significant pain, which might suggest a blood clot or area of intense bleeding. The nurses will also check your genital area especially as the catheter stays in for the first day. And they will check the feeling and circulation in your legs.

Some hospitals provide a device that cuffs around your legs and massages the surface so that circulation is improved. Clots can be an issue when you are not able to feel or move.

Once you have survived the first 24 hours, you can schedule more visitors. Recovery from natural childbirth and c-section are totally different. So when you schedule your visitors, make sure the visit is brief, that it doesn't occur when you are eating a meal, and you will not be nursing during the visit.

Most hospitals are really great at providing meals for you while you stay at the maternity ward. For our first meal my husband was able to order from the menu and it was complimentary but most of the other meals I just ordered as much extra food as possible so we could both eat for free. Sometimes I'd order extra French fries for my kids and I always kept plenty of juice and water bedside so that I would have it for them. Again, this is SURVIVAL. Do what you have to do to survive this hospital stay. Save as much money as you can and always look for ways that you can save more!

CHAPTER SIX
Bringing babies home
When the real work begins.

Okay, so you just had your moment. Your time in the
spotlight. Not only did many people visit you in the hospital,
even the nurses and health care workers couldn't keep out of
your room for a long enough period of time to let you sleep.
When they wheeled you out of the ob ward and into the
elevator to bring you to your car, those babies who were
positioned one on each arm made many people stop and look.
Twins attract attention. So get used to it. I still can't go to the
grocery store without allowing for extra time to shop.
Everyone loves twins.

But once you survive the first car ride home, and settle into
your favorite chair, reality has a tendency to sink in. You look
around, your house needs cleaning, your kids need a bath (if
you have other children), and the unknowns of life with twins
can make you feel overwhelmed. To make matters worse,
your twin belly is probably still fairly bloated from childbirth,
especially if you've had a c-section. There is so much to do
both inside and out of you, that you feel completely helpless.
But FEAR NOT. Help is on the way. It is called
ORGANIZATION....

It's time to get organized! There are three areas you must
learn to get organized in. The first is your mind. You must
organize the inside of you before you work on anything on the
outside.

The first area to organize is your mind. The mind is crucial to your future. How you approach your twin life now affects everything you face in the future. If you learn how to enjoy your double blessing and cherish all the moments you get to experience, you will feel so much better. But first you must fix the broken parts of your mind. Unfortunately because you've had double hormones raging through your body, the aftermath when all hormone levels attempt to return to normal can be a greater challenge than you've faced with previous pregnancies. But you will overcome and you will enjoy your new life-just relax, take a deep breath, and open your mind to the next several paragraphs.

First, you must learn to cry. So much of post-partum depression has been linked to hiding emotions. You are a woman. You need to cry when you feel like it. So let it out. Really. Watch a sad movie if you need help getting those tears out. It will make you feel so much better. Purposefully cry in front of your hubby. Let him know this is not going to be all flowers and sunshine. Agree that at any time you need to cry, that you can freely cry. And tell him what he needs to do to make you feel better. Hold you, wash the dishes, or deal with the kids...or maybe all three. God created man and woman as a unit together to help each other. We are to serve each other. That means when one person is down the other person needs to kick it in high gear. And now it's time for him to pay you back for your hard work. Really. Your husband needs to step up to the plate. Carrying those twins for 8-9 months was more work for your body than he will ever experience for himself. So husbands, it's time for payback.

And he will pay you back. Men are amazing. They have way more strength deep inside than any of us women ever thought they had.

The second area to organize is your environment. A clean house means so much when you have new babies in the home. You are going to have visitors and you will want a tidy house ON-DEMAND. Just like going to the channel and selecting a movie to watch on demand at any time, you want your house to be able to get cleaned on demand, too. That means the big cleanings get taken care of weekly and the tidying up is taken care of multiple times a day. If you are struggling to get the work done, consider hiring someone or asking friends and relatives to pitch in. Do not be afraid to recruit help. People want to help you. But, just like sometimes your husband can't read your mind, your friends and relatives can't read your mind either. So be vocal and be firm.

The third area to organize is your social life. Everyone will want to come and visit your twins. EVERYONE. And although it's nice to have an extra set of hands in the house, guests can seriously interfere with your ability to nurse, or take a nap, or just relax. So if you've scheduled some visitors to come and hold your babies, you need to organize their visit so you can get through it and feel so much better. Remember, they eventually leave and that's where the overwhelming emotions tend to kick in and catch you by surprise.

SURVIVING HOUSE VISITORS
First, decide what they can bring with them. That's right-bring with them. My visitors usually brought diapers or dinner or BOTH. We needed help especially extra diapers and food. Those were our basic needs. So we told all visitors to bring these items. And they didn't mind. People want to help but hear this…they aren't mind readers. They aren't mind readers. TELL THEM WHAT YOU NEED. Don't be shy and don't be embarrassed. You need help. So recruit it.

I had a rough time after delivery. The C-section was difficult and then I was hospitalized again for hypertensive crisis. Adding to the issues of my health, my 6 year old and 10 year old tested positive for influenza type H1N1 the day after I gave birth to my girls. My husband and I didn't have time to eat because we were taking care of everyone, running around disinfecting the house, wearing gloves and masks, isolating sick people from the healthy...it was horrible. We really didn't have time to cook. So most of our visitors brought dinner with them. That way we could feed the kids and ourselves when we got hungry. Once the first few weeks passed, we asked visitors to bring a pack of diapers with them. Because we were insistent on guests bringing diapers, we have only had to purchase three boxes (yes, boxes you will buy boxes) of diapers at about $35.00 each by the time the babies turned 6 months old! And honestly, as much as you think it's rude, it is not AT ALL. People don't know how to help but they WANT to help. So let them help YOU by telling them what YOU need. Otherwise they will just bring something you don't need. And how is that helping when they bring you what you don't need??? Think about it.

Second, only accept visitors when it's a good time for the babies. With two babies you must put them on a schedule. And with two babies you will find it easier to receive visitors when it's good for the babies' schedule, not for theirs. So set some visiting hours in your mind and stick to them. People are busy so give them choices on hours to visit. And if they ask why they can't visit any time, simply tell them you are bringing the babies to an appointment. Seriously it's NONE of their business so you don't owe them any explanation. I just found it more helpful to say I wouldn't be home because people will pop over anyways if they think you are there. On several occasions I wanted to hide my car for the day...really.

Third, get plenty of hand sanitizer and spray disinfectant. You will need to cleanse your home after visitors just in case they've brought any germs. Insist they wash their hands and use hand sanitizer. Germs are everywhere and when you have visitors these germs will come in on them. Literally thousands of germs can be brought in on people. So clean clean clean…it will keep your babies safer.

And lastly, do not allow small children over to see the babies. This is a big one. I know you want everyone to be able to visit with your new bundles but small children are infested with dangerous germs. They could be carrying around all kinds of dangerous germs and not show any symptoms of having any illness. If they hold the babies it's even worse because many of these germs are located inside their mouths and respiratory system. The mouth of a small child will be in closer proximity to the baby's mouth than that of an adult's. If they breathe on the babies they could get them sick. Babies have a sensitive immune system. They haven't lived long enough to get strong against germs and it takes years for their immunity to build. You can't expose them to a lot of germs.

Feeding two babies at once…it can be done and it can give you a much-needed break

The decision to breastfeed or formula feed is a tough one. Every mother has a right to decide what is best for her own babies. I breastfed all 6 of my previous children successfully so when I went to breastfeed my new twins, I thought it would be a breeze.

Boy was I wrong! I had such a struggle with breastfeeding. I searched online for help and tried everything the experts suggested to do. I pumped, I squeezed, and honesty I agonized in pain. Breastfeeding two was tough. Complicating matters I was scared to breastfeed them because I was on 600mg. of Beta Blockers and 35mg. of Calcium Channel Blockers to manage my Pregnancy Induced Hypertension. I feared that these drugs would enter their system. No matter what anyone else told me....

Looking back on those days, I wish I had just formula fed the twins in the first place. They are healthy, thriving, and developing perfectly and doing all this on formula. They aren't any more susceptible to colds and other viruses than my breastfed babies were. Actually now that they are 2 they've each only been sick once!! But for sake of you understanding that you are not a bad mom if you decide either way, I will take you back in time…to the beginning of my breastfeeding battle…and to the birth of my twins.

So there they were, gorgeous and identical, two healthy and happy blonde haired blue eyed newborn babies. It was time for them to eat and therefore time for me to assume the position to feed them. I still wasn't able to move my lower legs because of the anesthesia given to me in the C-section. So the nurses had to help me and hand me the babies to feed. I tucked pillows where they instructed me to tuck them. Cleared the room of all visitors and got ready for what I thought would be one of the greatest moments of my life.

Wrong. One of the early struggles in breastfeeding a newborn is keeping the baby attached to the breast. And one of the early pains in breastfeeding is when the baby continues to lose his/her latch on the nipple. OUCH!!! OUCH TIMES TWO!!!! It wasn't working out very well for me at all. At least not with two. So I placed one baby back in the crib, and attempted to feed them one at a time.

One at a time doesn't work either. First, you will constantly have a baby on the breast. Constantly. As soon as one baby is done nursing the other baby will need to be nursed. Once burped and both are changed, the cycle repeats itself again. Second, because you aren't feeding them at the same time your breasts wont produce enough milk to feed them both. And third, your milk will have an issue letting down because you will be tense from the baby in the crib crying in wait as you nurse his/her twin. One at a time is a complete disaster.

So I tried two at a time again. This time my husband came over to help. He had to keep one twin attached on one breast as I attached the other twin to the other breast. This worked for three minutes. But then the babies fell off the breast and when he put my breast back in one twin's mouth, I screamed bloody murder because the latch was off and I felt shooting pains radiate through my chest. I was done.

Then the wonderful nurses tried to help. This was a failure as well. They did the same thing my husband did by keeping one twin on one breast as I fed the other twin with the other breast. And the same thing happened. The nurses were much better at putting the baby back on the breast. But I felt like my privacy was being violated. And I wanted the nurses to leave the room so I could have alone time while nursing. Instead of it being an intimate moment between mom and babies, I felt like a science experiment.

Through trial and error, and unsuccessful feeding and pumping, I decided to let the babies have formula so that I didn't starve them to death. By the time I left the hospital, the babies were on both breast milk and formula. It wasn't my version of an ideal situation, but I knew that I couldn't compare my twin experience to any other singleton experience. Twins were different, in every way. And they made sure I knew it from very early on.

For the next several weeks breastfeeding was a battle. Not 24 hours after they released me from the hospital, I was rushed back into the OB ward in "hypertensive crisis". My blood pressure was shooting up and I felt horrible. For the next 3 days I had to stay in the hospital. I did it without my babies and husband. That experience felt like it would never end. I was scared and missed my twins. But I was at risk of dying from complications. And the nurses and doctors had to keep me calm.

They delivered blood pressure lowering drugs and altered my doses until they felt confident that I could leave the hospital and monitor my own blood pressure at home. But those three days in the hospital were days my milk was coming in. The babies weren't with me and every time I sat up to pump my breasts my blood pressure would shoot up high. My milk levels came in low, too low to sustain two other lives. I left the hospital confused and upset. But because I didn't want to raise my blood pressure any higher, I went home and gave up on the breastfeeding almost entirely, choosing only a few feedings a day to put the twins to the breast.

For the next six weeks I struggled to breastfeed my babies. I saw a lactation lady and she gave me absolutely no help. I left the appointment with a new breast pump, instructions on how to be a human cow, and the conclusion in my head that the lactation lady needed to quit talking about boobs all day. I rented that pump and didn't use it one time.

I quit the nursing quest permanently when the twins were seven weeks old. Between the fact that my milk hadn't come in well, the reality that I was probably on too may blood pressure lowering drugs to guarantee my twins' safety, and the overall exhaustion that I felt on all those drugs, I decided it was best to stick to formula. I felt like a failure.

To this day I still hear from people recommending I should've tried breastfeeding longer. I always respond with a smile and say, "you take out your boobs and feed them at the same time and let me know how that works for you"...in other words "be quiet"...you gotta love the unsolicited advice...

I am in no way advocating against breastfeeding, I just want you to understand that whatever you decide don't worry about making the wrong choice. The decision on how to feed your twins is a personal decision between you and the babies. No one else has the right to pressure you into deciding any different.

So onto the details about feeding your lovely twins.

Breastfeeding twins is tricky. If you've ever breastfed your infant, I'm sure one of the first positions you enjoyed was the lying down position, particularly in the middle of the night. Umm...well. This won't work with twins. It's impossible. The only positions where you can feed two babies simultaneously are the ones while you sit up and hold the babies. These are the double cradle or cross cradle hold, the football hold, the crisscross or front V hold, and the saddle or parallel hold.

- Double Cradle or Cross Cradle Hold: This position combines the football hold and a cradle hold. The babies lie across the mother with their bodies and feet pointing to the side, in the same direction. Moms' hands and arms cradle the babies' heads and upper back. One baby's legs extend under Mom's arm, as in the football hold. One baby's head may rest on the other's body.

- **Crisscross or Front-V Hold**: The babies' heads rest on Mom's forearms as her hands cradle their bodies from underneath. Their bodies cross on Mom's lap, with legs pointing in opposite directions.

- <u>Saddle or Parallel Hold:</u> The babies are upright, facing mom's chest. Best for older babies who are capable of sitting up.

- **Football Hold:** The babies' heads are positioned in front of mom's chest, with their bodies extending back. Mom's hands support both babies heads and her forearms support both babies' bodies. The legs can either fall under or outside mom's arms. The football hold works very well with infants, as there is more control of the babies' wobbly heads. This is also a very comfortable position for mothers who delivered via cesarean section.

Formula Feeding:

And of course, there's always formula. I think when I was a baby my mother fed me corn syrup and carnation instant milk. Well, alternatives to breast milk have come a long way. And formula today is extremely healthy for your infants. So if you have to wean, at whatever age, you know you have some great choices to bottle feed those babies.

Placing twins on the same schedule (which mine are on to this day) begins at feeding time. So you've put away the boobs, filled two bottles with formula, and it is time to bottle-feed times two. You need to feed them at the same time...which is super easy with a little creativity.

- ✓ GET HELP. Have someone take one twin while you feed the other twin. This is of course the easiest way. But it does require another human being to help.
- ✓ PROP. Okay I know...never prop a bottle. Well that isn't entirely true. If you are right there watching the propped bottles, there is nothing wrong with propping a bottle. If I hadn't propped bottles to get through formula feeding times two, I'm pretty sure I'd be in an insane asylum right now. Often the only time you will get to take a breather is when the twins are feeding. I would prop both bottles,

keep the twins in plain sight, and do other tasks like washing dishes while they were feeding. I never took my eyes off of them when they were feeding while propping. And neither should you.

✓ GET TWO HANDS INVOLVED. My favorite position was placing each twin on either side of me, head towards me, and bodies lined up outside of me. I was able to stick one bottle in each mouth, and feed both at the same time.

✓ PROP ONE WHILE HOLDING THE OTHER. This is great especially when you just don't have the energy to hold both. I suffered a lot with exhaustion while I was on my blood pressure meds. I simply didn't have the energy to feed both babies at the same time. So I would hold one baby and prop the other baby's bottle at feeding time. And for the next feeding, I'd switch who got propped and who got held.

The diaper changing system that works...

I thought I couldn't handle the expense of diapering two babies. So in my inexperience with twins, I assumed I could diaper my bundles with cloth, save money and help the environment. I put cloth diapers on my registry, I put in an order for some to be sent, but by a miracle of God none ever came. And I do mean miracle. Because God literally had to save me from myself. From my own delusion, let me explain by sharing with you the reality of diapering for two.

SURVIVING DIAPERS TIMES TWO
It isn't that much harder than diapering for one. Really. I change my babies on one of two surfaces. If I'm downstairs I change them on the changing table attached to the pac n play. I leave one twin in the bassinet of the pac n play while I change the first baby, and then when I'm done I switch positions and change the other baby.

I keep a garbage can handy right next to the pac n play and it has a handy diaper stacker attached to the side. If I'm upstairs I use the crib that has the changing table attached and I use the same routine as I use downstairs. One baby gets to hang out in the crib as I change the other one and then I switch babies when done. I keep a garbage can handy to toss the soiled diapers in, and I keep plenty of supplies within arms reach nearby.

I got very quick at diaper changes. I sometimes think I could win a speed contest for diapering.

But that is speed with disposable diapers. I grab them, use them, and throw them out. Laundry is challenging enough, as the twins get older, I couldn't imagine throwing diapers into the already overwhelming to do list for laundry. Also, when we are out and about, twins usually poop at the same time. So struggling with cloth diapers, carrying the soiled ones back home to pop in the washer, and trying to get rid of that awful smell times two that follows you around is a tall order for any new mom.

Life with twins is much easier to survive when you SIMPLIFY. For my husband and I it was a no brainer. Use the disposables and live in peace. But if you must use cloth, utilize the cloth with the Velcro straps, and consider using disposables when you are out. Purchase a minimum of 3 days worth of diapers for each child. And enjoy ☺

And here's the big diapering secret…when you put the babies on the same schedule, they will usually soil their diapers near the same time. For the first 6 months this is very true. Now I notice that sometimes I don't need to change them both at the same time, and now that they are older it's okay because I can pretty much change them anywhere I need to.

Looking back on my delusional days when I felt like getting cloth diapers to save money, I am thankful I didn't follow through on that idea. It is much easier to throw those diapers out and grab new ones. And I seriously have enough laundry to do on a daily basis anyways. I couldn't imagine adding more clothes to my already full hamper.

Sleeping through the night. It IS possible with two

It is very difficult to wake up several times in the middle of the night with two babies. This was a particular struggle for me because I rely on my ability to wake up at 5:30a.m. to write my books. Additionally I also pray and exercise before everyone wakes. So, for the first 6 weeks of my twin life, my schedule was crazy. My sleeping and waking times were all over the map! Complicating matters, I suffered with high blood pressure for several weeks after my twins were born. So sleep wasn't just convenient for me, it was critical to my survival. Recovery from childbirth relies heavily on the amount of sleep you get. So how the heck are you going to get sleep when you have TWO newborn babies?? It's time to learn the REAL WAY to make babies sleep through the night...

I have listed several things you can do to help your babies sleep through the night. However, you must make sure they can skip a feeding overnight so please ask your pediatrician if they are ready for this. Some babies do better than others. Some babies will need to feed overnight to prevent them from going back in the hospital, especially if they were born premature. My pediatrician didn't have a problem with mine sleeping through the night at six weeks but they are thriving and have never had a health issue. So check with your doctor about what your babies are ready for. And always follow his/her advice before you follow mine ☺.

1. Approach bedtime differently. Bedtime is not when your babies fall asleep, it   is when you decide to put them down for sleep. Your babies should not be in
    control of your sleep. You should dictate bedtime not your babies. Do you   wait until you are sleeping to go to bed? How about your other kids, do you   carry them to bed AFTER they fall asleep? No… so why should you do
    this   for the twins? Set a specific bedtime and stick to it regardless of whether   your bundles of joy are sleeping like babies or up like monsters!

2. Soothe their tummies. Babies are just like you or I. When their stomachs ache, they cannot sleep well. So the first thing you must do to set your babies up for sleeping through the night is get their feedings under control. If you are breastfeeding, avoid the trigger foods that can cause gas. If you are formula feeding, stick with ONE formula that doesn't cause their tummies to ache. Feed them right before you lay them down for the night. And make sure you burp them well.

3. Give them a solid routine around bedtime so they can learn that it is time to go to sleep. Do the same thing every night. Talk with the rest of the family and schedule a basic regimen you can use before you put them down for the night.

    a. Will you bathe them? If so, what time will you bathe them every night? If it's 8:00p.m., stick with that time and do it every night. What you are doing is essentially training them to understand it is time to relax and settle down for sleep.
    b. Will you rock them? My babies love the rocking chair. I can almost guarantee they will be sleeping within ten minutes of rocking. However, they didn't like it until they were about 3 months old. Find out if your little ones like to rock. And then

use the rocking chair for a specific amount of time every night. Stop rocking regardless of whether they are crying or not. If you've picked 15 minutes stick to the 15 minutes. Babies love routine.

c. Will you soothe them with sound? Reading to them or playing a lullaby c.d. in their nursery can help them understand it is time for bed. If they hear the same thing at the same time their brains, although small, will figure out that it is time to sleep. Babies brains work well and figure many things out before they are consciously aware of what they are doing. Choose a sleepy sound they can fall asleep to and stick with it.

d. Stick to the plan. If we deviate from the nighttime regimen we are usually headed for heartache. Just last night we watched a movie until 10:00p.m. The babies went to the crib on time but we didn't feed them their last bottle, they just fell asleep without it. And I was up several times overnight with a crying baby. I did not feed her but I did get up once and put her next to me to help her fall back to sleep. She was so upset that she gave herself the hiccups.

4. Reserve the crib for sleeping only at night. Although it is tempting to put them in their crib every time they sleep, this can get confusing for an infant. If you reserve the crib for overnight sleeping only they will associate their crib with sleeping overnight. Learn to place them in other areas like a pac-n-play or bassinet when they zonk out during the day.

5. Get them out of your room. I had 6 babies before my twins came into the world, and I always had a cradle or bassinet set up in my room by my bedside for those overnight wakings. With the twins, we had no choice but to place them in the nursery to sleep because there simply wasn't enough room to put two cradles or

bassinets by our bedside. Best thing I ever did. Because with my previous babies I would wake up for the smallest sound or movement, unaware that I was making the likelihood that the baby would sleep through the night ten times worse! Don't be afraid that you won't hear them wake up. You will. Keep your doors open and cut off all extra sound. You want to train them to quit waking up in the middle of the night which means they need to be in a separate room because as long as they are by your bedside they will think of food and wake up to feed. It is especially hindering to your success if you are still breastfeeding as they will smell your milk and wake up.

6. Get in a routine of putting them in their crib awake. This is possible with twins. Your babies like each other and are soothed by each other's company. When you place them down for the night, do it while they are awake. Allow them to fall asleep on their own. You will find they are quite different from other babies, as they feel less scared because they have each other. This is a great advantage with twins. You will usually hear some crying and at times that crying may get louder, but if you stick to this routine your twins will eventually surrender to sleep. And you will finally get some much-needed zzzs.

7. Consider putting the twins in the same crib together. Our twins are 6 months old. They roll over, push off, and try so hard to crawl. Right now when we discover them in their crib in the morning, we don't know what we will find. Usually one is on top of the other's arm, or one has the other by her hair. We have another crib to put together but we don't have the heart to separate them right now. They love to sleep in the same crib together and this is particularly helpful when you are trying to get them to sleep through the night. You will know when it is time to separate them but while you are training them

to sleep through the night, having them in the same crib together is helpful.

8. Lower the lights and the noise at the same time every night. We have a household of 8 with 4 of the most rambunctious boys you will ever meet. The noise level in my home can get quite loud so we have a set time every night for the world to quiet down. We dim the lights, lower the televisions, and either send the boys outside or in their rooms. When your household quiets down at the same time every night it helps your babies settle down too.

9. Consider getting a fish tank with bright colors to put in their nursery bedside. My babies love the fish tank. We have a saltwater aquarium with brightly colored clownfish and bright live rock. It isn't very expensive to maintain and the twins love to watch the fish. If they are struggling to get to sleep at night the fish tank will create enough of a diversion that they will drift away to sleep in no time once the fish catch their attention.

10. Turn off the baby monitors and shut the doors. Now it's time to get serious. As much as it probably breaks your heart at even the thought of ignoring your crying infants, this is crucial in helping them learn to sleep through the night. But the first thing you must do is prepare yourself to ignore their cries for help. I had to recruit my husband to put the twins to bed at night. He does this every night because if I do it, I will quickly scoop them back up once they start crying. We had to shut off the baby monitors and shut our bedroom door and their nursery door. So once all of this is done, we can normally catch some sleep and if they do wake through the night for a short period of time, we won't wake up to get them. If they are up for a longer period of time or their cries get serious, we will

wake up and peek in on them. No one has ever cried to death, at least I couldn't find real evidence of this happening. So rest assured, your babies will be fine if you let them cry it out a little.

11. And finally, do not pick them up if they wake up during the night except in cases of emergency. Emergencies include, spit up, soiled diapers, or leaking diapers. These warrant a wake up and an urge to change the baby. But other than emergencies, you should leave your waking infant in the crib until it is time to get up for the day. If you pick them up and cuddle them-or worse case scenario-FEED THEM to get them back to sleep, I guarantee they will wake up again the following night. Babies are super smart. Be smarter than them by keeping them in the crib through the whole night.

I hope you will implement the tips I've provided in this section. Once you are able to sleep a solid night through without waking to feed babies your life will slowly return to normal. Well, as normal as normal can be with twins. To this day there are nights when I can hear the twins fussing in the crib at 2a.m. I can't hear them unless I get up to use the bathroom. But I smile and avoid opening the nursery door. I know that if I dare open that and go to their rescue, they will learn to wake up in the middle of the night again to feed. The risk of starting that scenario all over again is too great and so I just quietly go back to bed and pray that they fall back asleep. The babies need a good night's sleep as much as you do. A lot of their growing happens when they are asleep. A baby who sleeps through the night early is usually a healthier baby. So as tough as it can be to ignore those cries or shut off that nursery monitor, in the end it is much better for you and the babies!

SURVING SEPERATION

Ugh! This is my least favorite section of the book. I don't even want to write it. But it is part of the twin experience so I have to include it. One of the hardest things for me was separating my twins into two different cribs. They love sleeping in the same crib together. And I spent many nights trying to calm very fussy babies as we attempted to separate them.

If you have your twins sleeping in separate cribs then you don't need to read this section. Congratulations! If you hadn't figured it out by now, twins love to be together. They have a sense when their other half is around them. If I put my twins in separate rooms they are never as happy as if I keep them side-by-side. This is true in the overnight hours as well. But eventually they will need to separate beds. Even if they choose to hang out in their twin's bed when they are older, you must provide the healthy environment now to encourage separate sleeping.

A few weekends ago my husband set up the second crib. I choked back my tears. It seemed logical to him to put up the other crib. For me I felt like it was cruel and I didn't want to do it. So I left the nursery and went downstairs to busy myself with dismantling the Christmas tree as he tinkered upstairs with the crib. It shouldn't have been a big deal but it was to me. I didn't want to separate the twins because they were so happy sleeping together. In the hospital they would cry and cry until they were placed in the same crib together. At home, they had never slept apart.

As a child I used to share a bedroom with my brother. I never minded being in the same room with him, although we fought a lot. I always found comfort in him being in the same room with me as I slept. Your twins are feeling the same comfort with each other. They shared months inside together as they were developing in the pregnancy. They love to be together and will probably never want to be apart-until the teenage years hit ☺.

But my husband kept putting the crib together, regardless of my protests. I wanted to vomit. Everything was perfect with the girls. They had been sleeping through the night for months. The twins slept for 11 hours straight every night. They woke up every day in the best mood! Why the heck would we risk ruining that now?

Separating your twins can be quite a challenge. I know you are probably thinking 'what's the big deal? It's just two beds…' Well, that's what my husband thought too. But then the problems began.

The first overnight they slept well. I put the moodier one in the old crib and chose to put my more content and laid back one in the new crib. They slept about 9 hours. Which was a little shorter than usual. But when they woke up, it was a whole different story.

They woke up screaming bloody murder. At first I thought maybe they both had sore tummies from something they ate, but they hadn't eaten any new baby food the night before. We changed them and brought them downstairs, just like we always do because twins love routine. Instead of smiling and delighting in seeing us, they were inconsolable until we put bottles in their mouths. It was horrible. But we didn't dare back down…not yet anyways. We went through the day and put them in separate cribs again for the overnight hours.

The second night Brooke, my moodier twin, was placed in the new crib. She woke up overnight several times but it wasn't too big of a cry so I just let her cry it out alone in bed. She woke up very early the next morning and was so tired. Both twins didn't seem like their normal happy selves. As a matter of fact, their entire schedule was wacked out. One would sleep while the other one was up practically the entire day. I figured I could get them back in routine the next day as the kids went to school and my husband went to work and it would just be the three of us at home.

The third night was a nightmare. And as I'm writing this I want you to understand that I am sharing these struggles with you so I can demonstrate the challenges we faced with our girls. You might not have any of these challenges. Your twins may love to sleep in their own crib. I am providing my story as kind of a "worst case scenario" so you can learn tips on how to overcome the dilemma if your twins don't want to separate.

Overnight on the third night Brooke again woke up. Only this time she was screaming bloody murder. I let her cry for over an hour before I got her up and put her in bed with me. She was upset, trying to catch her breath, but fell back asleep. I put her back in her crib (the new one) and she woke right up and resumed the inconsolable screaming.

I literally sat up for hours that night. Brooke was up for about 4 hours. I didn't dare feed her a bottle or rock her back to sleep. I knew I had to let her fight it out inside of herself. It was very difficult to let her but I did. The next day things got weird. Really weird.

The twins were not happy. For the first day since birth the girls were absolutely miserable. No smiles ran across their faces when they saw others in passing which was not normal for them. They are usually the showstoppers when I'm out. Their smiles radiate joy to everyone they meet. Not today, not with these two. They looked devastated. Their napping schedule was off too...way off. I decided I'd had enough and I was contemplating putting them together in the same crib again. And so I put the two in the jogging stroller and hit the local fitness trail to get some fresh air and clear my head. I was thinking about reuniting them in the same crib and felt like I might damage them if I never allow them to sleep in separate cribs. Almost as if by fate, I ran into a lady who I had seen exercising several times over the past two years. We always smiled at each other in passing but had never officially met. She stopped us and took a look at the twins. Her name was Maria. She had aunts who were twins. She loves twins.

I told her about the overnight plight we were having, apologizing for my twins' grumpy attitudes and explained how the separation thing wasn't working out for us. "I understand completely", she responded, she spoke with a Jamaican accent.

"Really?" I couldn't believe what I was hearing. But I wanted to hear more so I listened intently to her words.

"Yes, my twin aunts don't like to be apart either. As a matter of fact they still live together and they are both in their sixties. They tried to have boyfriends and live apart but they don't do well away from each other. So one would break up with her boyfriend, then the other one would break up with hers...then they would be together again and be happy." She smiled at Brooke. She gave her a smile as if she was thanking her for visiting and sharing.

Well, that was confirmation for me. I decided I wasn't going to force them to be apart. And I was going to ease them into separate sleeping instead of throwing it on them all at once. I decided that I'd rather the girls separate completely when they are ready. So I put Brooke and Esther together in the same crib that night. And they slept like they always had before. I peeked in the crib on them and saw they were sleeping so peacefully. The joy had returned. And I knew that I had not failed but rather I had triumphed as a twin mom because I valued their comfort and happiness over everyone else's opinion to separate the two of them. I decided I would let them sleep separately a few days a week to start. And just leave it at that. For as long as was necessary.

There are so many things that science does not understand about twins. As a science major, the only things we were taught about twins were the different types of twins and how they both share the same time in the uterus before entering the world.

Identical twins are clones of each other. Fraternal twins can be as different as night and day in appearance. But whether you have twins developing from one egg or two, they share many commonalities. Twins love to be together. They love to touch each other and they find comfort in being within a few inches of each other. Science cannot determine why this is. But I have.

It's love. They learned to love each other months before they took their first breath. When I was pregnant with Esther and Brooke only one sonogram showed them not face to face and it was at twelve weeks. Every single sonogram from 13 weeks on showed the girls interacting with each other and playing together. They loved to lie in many different positions, taking up as much room as possible inside, but their faces were always aligned up perfectly.

Sometimes we would marvel at how they looked like they were communicating, like they had their own way of sharing their world with the other twin. And of course that was why I ended up having a c-section delivery. They didn't want to leave my body and Twin A did not cooperate with my uterus and its two weeks of labor to try to get the babies to come out. Her plan was never to head for the exit because she didn't know she would see her sister again on the other side. No wonder they didn't like sleeping in separate cribs!

But as cute as it was, I knew I had to conquer this separate cribs thing. But like every single milestone with twins this was only a matter of time. Eventually around 14 months old, they started to fight physically with each other. And a few times I caught Esther on top of Brooke's head in the crib. That was all we needed to separate them and keep them separated. They are 2 now. And we just put their cribs together again. So I guess I haven't conquered the sleeping separate thing. As they are sleeping side by side once again.

One day they will be big enough to do their own thing. When I move them into toddler beds the girls will be able to decide for themselves if they'd like to sleep apart or together. But what I'm finding out is that twins are usually behind the curve on these things. Battling with two toddlers to stay in the toddler beds is a living nightmare. And so far, we haven't tried it!

Section three, getting back to "normal"

CHAPTER SEVEN
Getting your body back
How to get rid of your twin belly, for real.

First of all to enter this chapter of the book you need to be ready to be real. Read this after the baby comes and follow the advice I'm providing. My expertise is in this area. I've been as large as 275 pounds and as small as 130 pounds. I've gained and lost weight several times corresponding with every pregnancy. I'm also experienced as a Certified Personal Trainer for 8 years, holding a Personal Trainer certificate by one of the top 2 certifying boards in the world. I've worked in the fitness business regularly for 17 years and managed facilities for over 5. I studied for a degree in nutrition. And I have a Bachelor's of Science Degree in Exercise and Sports Science.

And just like I couldn't write this book about twin survival until I had experienced twins, no one can write a book on weight loss until they've succeeded themselves in losing weight. There are many misconceptions out on the market and countless myths that circulate the weight loss business, that you must have experience in successfully losing weight before you can really help others. Unfortunately there is so much misinformation on the market it is difficult to write the truth and have people follow it.

For whatever reason people like to be sold on the latest weight loss gimmick because it is endorsed by a celebrity or promises unreal super fast results.

However, celebrities get paid BIG BUCKS to endorse products. And that weight loss method they 'swear by' is only important to them because it put quite a few extra dollars in their pocket. I am not a celebrity. I am a weight loss EXPERT. I've taken a lifetime of experience and education to compile the following section so that you can be successful in losing weight. I've also included expertise by fitness professionals in this section. So they, too, can share their experiences with you. Bottom line…if you want results follow the system and you will get them. And if you don't want results, complain and continue to sit on the couch and eat junk food. And that brings us to the most important first step. Make a choice to lose weight. And continue every day to turn that choice into a lifetime commitment.

SURVIVING WEIGHT LOSS

First, you must commit to your weight loss journey. Commitment is the most important key to weight loss success. Yes, it is literally all under control of your mind. And it is a daily choice. Every day you must wake up and think of what you can do better to lose weight…every single day. Maybe it's getting a better workout in than you did the last time you trained, maybe it's saying no to certain foods, or maybe it's a combination of both. Commitment is key and without it you will not be successful.

Second, you must analyze your current state of health. Are you ready for this? Has your doctor cleared you for fitness? Are you experiencing any pain leftover from the childbirth? Perform a head to toe check of your body and determine if you are ready to begin a training regimen. This program starts out slow and is progressive. So if you can walk a mile without pain, you can start the program. Just make sure your doctor has cleared you to resume to normal activity. If he/she hasn't yet, don't worry. You will be cleared soon. And you can always work on your diet while you wait!

Third, determine where you are going to start working out. Do you have exercise equipment in the home? Or are you an outside person? Do you need to go to a gym or other fitness facility to get your workouts in? My recommendation is to start out slow. Real slow. Plan to do a short walk first as it will take several weeks to get up enough endurance to exercise long enough for weight loss, especially if you've been on bed rest or are recovering from a c-section. It took me four months of very light workouts to get me fit enough to exercise long enough for weight loss results. So be patient and be smart.

Fourth, determine what exercise 'hour' you will work out. This is probably going to be decided on by what you are going to do with the babies. If they are still waking through the night, you will want to take them with you. Your exercise "hour" will probably need to be a flexible time when the babies are awake and you won't be able to sleep anyways. Or if you are really brave you could get up earlier than the babies and exercise for the hour without them. I wake up at 5:00a.m. every day to get my workouts in. But when I was beginning my workout regimen, I had a difficult time getting up early even once a week. So I took my walk, my exercise hour, mid-morning with the babies in the stroller. Don't overdo or overachieve when you are starting out. Remember that you are in this for life and you have plenty of time to build your speed and distance. Right now you are laying the foundation for success. So you need to do what works for you and the babies. Choose a time and place that works around the babies schedule. As you get stronger and more confident you will be able to adjust your workout time.

Fifth, choose your fat burn exercise you will do on a daily basis. This could be biking, walking, rollerblading, jogging, aerobics class either at the health club or at home, swimming, etc. Find out what works for you. I suggest to my clients to think back on their childhood and determine what type of exercise they enjoyed when they were kids. I was a bike rider. And still love riding my bike as much today as I did when I was 10. So my first choice is biking. What did you like when you were younger? Maybe that's what you need to do today to be successful in losing weight. Have fun with your exercise choice. Drive to the water and push the stroller on the sidewalk alongside the waves. Or stay at home and put your favorite exercise d.v.d. in the player. Do what makes you enjoy your time exercising. You will be in it for the long haul so you must make sure you enjoy it.

And finally, Sixth, Write it down! Keep an exercise and food log. This is critical for success. You can write your workouts and diet down in a notebook, download an exercise and nutrition tracker app on your phone, or have one of your kids keep a log for you. Whatever works for you-do it. I look back on my fitness app and see that just 3 months ago I was walking a mile in almost an hour and stopping four times during that hour. Today I can jog 5 or 6 miles and ride my bicycle 20 miles at a time. I didn't get to where I am now all in one day, of course. I gradually progressed as I got stronger and I recovered from the childbirth. And that log that you might think is a pain to do will keep track of your success so when you are having days where you feel you can't do any more, you will have ability to look back on how far you've come!

And it all counts towards calories burned. Here is a list of various exercises and the calories that are burned during them. Keep note of these and if you are crunched for time but need a good calorie burn opt for the exercises that will burn the most calories in the least amount of time.

Activity (1-hour duration) Weight of person and calories burned (chart taken from mayoClinic.com)

	160 lbs(73 kg)	200 lbs(91 kg)	240 lbs(109 kg)
Aerobics, high impact	533	664	796
Aerobics, low impact	365	455	545
Aerobics, water	402	501	600
Backpacking	511	637	763
Basketball game	584	728	872
Bicycling, < 10 mph, leisure	292	364	436
Bowling	219	273	327
Canoeing	256	319	382
Dancing, ballroom	219	273	327
Football, touch or flag	584	728	872
Golfing, carrying clubs	314	391	469
Hiking	438	546	654
Ice skating	511	637	763
Racquetball	511	637	763
Resistance training	365	455	545
Rollerblading	548	683	818

Rope jumping		
861	1,074	1,286
Rowing, stationary		
438	546	654
Running, 5 mph		
606	755	905
Running, 8 mph		
861	1,074	1,286
Skiing, cross-country		
496	619	741
Skiing, downhill		
314	391	469
Skiing, water		
438	546	654
Softball or baseball		
365	455	545
Stair treadmill		
657	819	981
Swimming, laps		
423	528	632
Tae kwon do		
752	937	1,123
Tai chi		
219	273	327
Tennis, singles		
584	728	872
Volleyball		
292	364	436
Walking, 2 mph		
204	255	305
Walking, 3.5 mph		
314	391	469

Weight loss is not that complicated. You just have to take a few minutes every day and think about what you are going to do differently to lose weight. One pound of fat lost is equal to 3,500 extra calories burned. If your goal is to lose between one and two pounds a week, I recommend striving to exercise an additional 500 calories a day to burn and combine it with an additional 500 calorie deficit of what you normally eat. In other words, BURN 500 and SAY NO to 500.

BURN 500 and SAY NO to 500.

So...to summarize the steps.

STEP ONE-Commit to daily exercise
STEP TWO-Assess your current health status
STEP THREE-Determine where you will work out
STEP FOUR-Determine your exercise 'hour'
STEP FIVE-Determine what you will do for your exercise
STEP SIX-Keep a log of your workouts and diet

After you've spent several weeks getting your cardiovascular exercise in, it's time to get your muscles stronger by building them. As those babies get older you will need to have stronger muscles, particularly in your arms. I still hold my twins one on each arm. And they weigh in at 26 pounds each! I couldn't have handled carrying them at their current weight a year ago. I had to get stronger as they got heavier. So just like your daily exercise, you must commit to a weight-training program that will progressively strengthen your muscles while your little bundles of joy get heavier and more difficult to handle.

And an added bonus to weight training is that one extra pound of muscle burns an additional 6.5 calories per hour according to the latest data on exercise physiology. Contrasting that a pound of body fat burns only 1.2 calories per pound per hour. So if you lose 10 pounds without adding muscle onto your frame, you actually LOWER your metabolism by at least 288 calories less burned every day but if you replace that tissue loss with 10 pounds of lean muscle tissue, your scale won't budge but you have increased your metabolism and can burn an extra 1,272 calories to that 10 pound body fat loss. So, yeah, weight training is a BIG deal. There are other benefits of weight training. These include…

- Weight training creates an increased after burn when you train - High intensity strength training can burn extra calories for hours after you have finished with your workout.

- Weight training prevents the loss of lean body mass that happens from dieting and aging

- Weight training changes your body composition, which shapes your body and keep you healthy

- Weight training strengthens bones and helps prevent osteoporosis.

- Weight training keeps you strong and active as you get older which helps stave off depression

- Weight training improves coordination, balance and helps prevent injuries

I hope I have convinced you to begin a weight-training regimen. If you have trouble getting started and need some assistance, check out other resources in addition to this workout that will be able to give you the added support you need. I highly recommend hiring a personal trainer, even if it's only for a short period of time. Trainers are experts in fitness and the right one can assist you in getting into a smart workout routine custom tailored for your body. A trainer will also be able to tell you about any postural distortions you have and will be able to give you stretching techniques to help improve your overall posture. These postural distortions eventually will cause other problems within your body if they are not corrected. If you have a body that is not aligned properly it will cause an abnormal pull on your muscles and ligaments and tendons that will create an additional load and strain on your joints. This additional abnormal pull and strain is what causes osteoarthritis and injury when you are older. Hiring a good personal trainer and having him/her help you with your posture is an invaluable investment in your future.

There are also various workout videos available that you can rent and purchase. Some of these videos are just for aerobic workouts while others have weight training and stretching. Choose a video that is fun and one that you will want to watch over and over again. Purchase weights in increments to go with the videos so that you can increase strength over time. And of course the Internet is a great resource as well. There are ways to recruit extra help for your weight training program so as I always have told my clients-NO EXCUSES GET ACTIVE AND STAY ACTIVE.

SURVIVING THE WORKOUT

You should begin this workout/weight training regimen about one day a week. Your goal is to get up to two days. This is a starter routine with progressions.

If the beginning set and rep recommendations are too easy for you, progress to more sets or reps or both. A rep is one complete movement of the exercise. A set is the reps completed without rest. For example...2 sets of 12 reps of a squat would be 12 squat motions repeated without rest. Then rest for 30 to 60 seconds. And repeat squats for another 12 reps. Rest between the sets as long as you need up to one minute. If you progress too soon or have pain, you can always back track to where you were before. As always, get permission from your doctor before beginning the routine in this book. And remember...weight training is a lifelong endeavor. Rushing it could bring you a lifelong injury.

Total Body Strength Routine for After Babies

Included is a 45-minute strength routine you can do in the comfort of your own home.

<u>Squat-</u>*2 sets of 10-12. Progress to 4 sets of 15*
Description-
Stand with feet about hip distance apart and parallel. Feet should be lined up with your shoulders. Dumbbells should be at your sides.
Bend at knees and stick glutes out behind you.
Keep back straight and the weight in your heels as you lower towards ground, mimicking sitting in a chair, arms at sides.
Sometimes it's helpful if you do squats in front of a chair.
As you return to fully standing, squeeze your glutes.
Progress to Squat Press
Same motion as above, but as you return to fully standing and squeeze your glutes, take dumbbels at shoulders and press towards the ceiling. Return back to shoulders to repeat entire movement.

Deadlift-2 *sets of 10-12. Progress to 4 sets of 15*
Description-
Stand with feet hip distance apart and parallel as you did with the squat.
With straight legs and back, hinge at hips while reaching arms down toward floor.
The dumbbells should be in front of your shins at bottom of movement. If that hurts at all in the back, only lower the weights to knee height.
Return to starting position by squeezing glutes.

Progress to Deadlift Row
Same motion as above, but as you bring the dumbbells to bottom of the movement, then engage your back and pull the dumbbells up by squeezing your shoulder blades together and rowing back with your elbows. Return to bottom of deadlift exercise and then return to starting position by squeezing glutes.

Bicep Curls-2 *sets of 10-12. Progress to 4 sets of 10-12*
Description-
Stand with feet shoulder width apart and parallel.
With dumbbells in hands, arms at sides, palms up
Lift weights up by bending elbows and squeezing biceps.
Keep elbows tucked into sides.
Return to start and repeat.

Progress to Curl Press
As you squeeze biceps and keep elbows tucked into sides, rotate your hands to point palms in front of you and away. Keep abs tight as you now press dumbbells up towards ceiling. Return weights to about shoulder height, rotate to face palms towards you.
Return to start position and repeat.

Overhead Dumbbell Presses-2 *sets of 10-12. Progress to 4 sets of 10-12*

Description

Stand with feet hip distance apart and parallel, abs drawn in.
With dumbbells in hands, arms bent out to sides at 90-degree angle with knuckles up, hands at shoulders.
Press weights overhead, keeping abs tight.
Lower weights slowly and return to start position and repeat.

Progress to Overhead Dumbbell Press standing on one leg for Balance during whole movement. Switch leg that you stand on for each set

While doing above exercise, stand on one foot with other foot placed near ground. Remain on one foot through entire set. Switch standing foot for each set.
Progress to keeping foot towards knee with knee and hip bent.

Triceps Extension, right arm then left arm-2 Sets of 10-12. Progress to 4 sets of 10-12

Description

Stand with feet shoulder width apart, right hand on hip
Reach left arm straight up holding dumbbell
Bend arm at elbow and drop weight slowly to just before 90 degrees
Squeeze tricep to slowly straighten back up.
Repeat on left arm for full set then switch to right arm. Once you complete both sides you have completed one set.

Progress to Tricep Dips off Couch or Bench

Stand in front of couch or bench facing away.
Place your hands on front edge of couch or bench.
Slowly lower yourself down in a sitting position until you've reached a 90-degree bend in elbows.
Press yourself back up through the triceps until your elbows extend almost fully.
To make this movement easier, bring your feet closer to the couch or bench.
To make this movement more challenging, bring your feet further out from the couch or bench.

Assisted Push Ups-2 *Sets of 10 reps. Progress to 3 sets of 12 reps*

With body facing floor bend at knees place hands on floor in line with shoulders.

Squeeze your back slightly to stabilize your shoulders.

Assuming a nice push up position with abs held in forming a straight line from knees to shoulders (at an angle) bend at elbows bringing your chest towards the floor.

When you get close to the floor, push back up using your chest.

Return to beginning and repeat.

Progress to Regular Push Ups

Same movement as above but place feet on floor instead of knees.

Dumbbell Back Rows-2 *Sets of 10 reps. Progress to 4 sets of 15 reps*

Stand hinged forward at hip, keeping back straight and abs pulled in.

Bring dumbbells to your sides, reaching to the floor.

Bend at elbows to pull weights up toward chest, squeeze shoulder blades together as you bring weights back in a rowing manner.

Return to beginning and repeat. This movement should be slow and controlled throughout.

ABS

Plank *First hold for 5 seconds 12 reps. Progress to more time holding and less reps to eventually get to 60 second holds 3 reps with 1-minute rest in between.*

Lie face down

Push up off floor onto elbows and toes. Keep elbows in line with your shoulders.

Keeping a straight line, hold the position with a flat back throughout the exercise.
Slowly lower yourself to ground, rest, and repeat.

Hip Bridge-*As many as you can do for 60 seconds at least 2 second hold in top of movement.*
Description-
Lie on your back on a mat on the floor.
Place both hands by sides, knees bent.
Keep weight in heels, squeeze glutes and push hips up towards ceiling so body is in one line from knees to shoulders.
Return to starting position and repeat.

Reverse Curls-*2 Sets of 20. Progress to as many as you can do!*
Lie on floor on back with both hands behind head.
With legs bent, pull knees in towards head.
Movement should be minimal, only a few inches.
Return to start and repeat.
Progress the movement by lifting shoulders off floor into a crunch and hold throughout the movement.

Basic Crunch-*2 Sets of 20. Progress to as many as you can do!*
Lie on floor on back with both hands behind head. Knees bent.
Keep lower back on floor.
Lift shoulders off floor, engaging your core muscles.
Return to start and repeat.
This move can be done at same time as reverse curls to make it more difficult.

Right Oblique Crunch-*1 Set of 15. Progress to 2 sets of 12 reps*
Lie on floor on back with right hand behind head. Knees bent.

Place left hand on right side of stomach.
Lift right shoulder off floor.
Bring right elbow towards left knee.
Return to start and repeat.

Left Oblique Crunch-1 *Set of 15. Progress to 2 sets of 12 reps*

Lie on floor on back with left hand behind head. Knees bent.
Place right hand on left side of stomach.
Lift left shoulder off floor.
Bring left elbow towards right knee.
Return to start and repeat.

Crossover Crunch-1 *Set of 15. Progress to 2 sets of 12 reps*

Lie on floor with both hands behind head, knees bent.
Lift right shoulder off floor and lift leg off floor.
Bring right elbow to left knee.
Repeat on other side and alternate the movement.

Superman-1 *Set of 10 reps. Progress to 3 sets of 12 reps*

Lie face down on your stomach with arms and legs extended.
Keep your neck in a neutral position.
Keeping your arms and legs straight but not locked and torso stationary, lift your arms and legs up toward the ceiling to form an elongated "u" shape with your body. Back should arch up and arms and legs should lift off the floor.
Hold for 2 to 5 seconds and then lower back down to starting position.
Repeat.

NUTRITION AND ABOLISHING THE DIET MYTHS

Before beginning the section on nutrition, I wanted to address some of the most popular workout and dieting myths out there on the market. Because my expertise is in the science behind exercise and nutrition, I would like to take time out and apply science to the most popular myths so that you can understand the truth behind the lies.

Myth #1-CARBS MAKE YOU FAT

Carbohydrates are the body's main energy source. Overeating calories makes you fat. It's a simple case of output vs. input. Take in more calories than you burn and you will get fat. Burn more calories than you consume and you will lose weight. It's completely scientific and no fad diet will ever change the science.

Myth #2-CUTTING CARBOHYDRATES WILL HELP YOU LOSE WEIGHT

Where the myth may have come from-people tend to overeat carbohydrates and under exercise. This myth probably began from a heart doctor who placed his clients on a low-carbohydrate diet for their heart health and discovered the clients were losing lots of weight. There are several issues with this scenario.

First, the patients he placed on this low carbohydrate diet were primarily elderly. As we get older, our bodies need less food. Less fats, less proteins, and less carbohydrates. So these patients needed less calories and when they reduced their carbohydrate intake, they reduced their total calorie intake, resulting in body fat loss. In other words, it helped reduce their total calorie intake because they weren't that hungry to replace the calorie loss with a high fat or high protein food.

Second, these patients needed less energy to get through their day. The reduced carbohydrate intake did not adversely affect their energy levels. So they didn't overeat the foods they were allowed to consume. Simply put, they lost weight because they took in less calories than they consumed.

> *Body check-cutting out carbohydrates will drain you of the energy you need for workouts. When you are drained of energy you will overeat calories in proteins and fats to replenish your energy stores.*

Smart check-make the carbohydrates work better for you by replacing refined sugar products with whole-grain alternatives. Replace white rice with brown rice. Replace white bread with whole-grain breads. Replace white pasta with whole-wheat pasta. And find low calorie alternatives to the snacks you grab. Eat popcorn instead of chips. Replace quick to grab carbohydrates with fruits and vegetables.

Myth #3-IF I SKIP MEALS I WILL NOT LOSE WEIGHT BECAUSE MY BODY WILL GO INTO STARVATION MODE Where the myth may have come from-people tend to keep lousy records. So a person who is skipping meals is probably not writing what they eat down. Have you ever seen a person who is actually starving? Their bodies are super skinny and they usually have a protruding abdomen because of lack of proper nutrients. In contrast, people who claim to have dropped their body into starvation mode are just as overweight as they've ever been. This is probably due to a drop in metabolism COMBINED with a really horrible diet.

Body check-When you drop your calorie intake over a period of time and you lose weight, your body's metabolism does adjust. It will burn at a slightly lower rate. However, if you are continuing to restrict calories you will continue to lose weight. Starvation mode is not some phenomenon that shows up in the body to hold onto excess body weight. It is simply a person not supplying his/her body with a steady supply of nutrients that will over time result in a slightly lower metabolism. But a person will lose weight if they are truly starving themselves. This starvation mode was just a fake tool people used to sell weight loss books. Period. AND IT SOLD THEM.

Smart check-do not ever skip meals. You want your metabolism to burn as efficiently as possible while you are losing body fat. Spike your metabolism by getting regular exercise and supplying your body with a steady supply of nutrients. Choose foods that raise your metabolism. Like high fiber and low fat foods. And by all means if you are hungry...eat. Just be smarter about what you eat when those hunger pangs strike.

Myth #4-FAT MAKES YOU FAT
Where the myth may have come from-I read a book that mentioned this several times. It was a weight loss book and the author made the stark claim that "fat makes you fat." It is a fact that per gram dietary fats have over twice as many calories as carbohydrates and proteins. Fat weighs in at 9 calories per gram while carbohydrates and proteins weigh in at 4 calories per gram each. Eating lots of fat will increase your total caloric intake. If you are limiting fats you drop your total caloric intake. However if you apply science to the myth, you will see that fats are vital for a healthy and functioning body.

Body check-While limiting your fat intake is always a healthy method to lose weight, zeroing in on fat and avoiding its' consumption entirely is a very bad idea. Every person needs fats. There are essential body fats that are crucial to perform functions within a body's metabolism. Every single cell within the body contains essential fatty substances in their membranes. Fat is a great source of energy, particularly when one is exercising at a steady moderate rate. Fat cushions organs and insulates the body. Fat generates heat. Hormones rely on fat to produce them and protect them and fats aid in the absorption and transportation of several vital fat-soluble nutrients and vitamins.

Smart Check-Because one gram of fat contains over twice as many calories as other nutrients it is a great idea to limit your consumption of total fat per day to lower your total caloric intake. Try to limit your intake of saturated and trans fat to help lower the "bad" fats in your daily diet. These "bad" fats have been linked to several problems including heart disease and coronary artery disease. They raise the cholesterol levels in your blood and are linked to all the diseases associated with higher cholesterol amounts. Limit them and you greatly reduce the health risk associated with these fats. While choosing your foods and choosing your fats, opt for polyunsaturated and monounsaturated fats as these fats increase your 'good' cholesterol levels within the body. Increasing your intake of these fats can greatly reduce the risks associated with the intake of the "bad" fats. Good sources of monounsaturated fats include olives, olive oil, canola oil, avocados, peanut oil, peanuts and most other nuts. Polyunsaturated fats can be divided into two main categories, omega-3 and omega 6 fatty acids. Good sources of omega-3s include oily fish (salmon, tuna, herring, swordfish), canola oil, soy oil, and any spreads made from these oils.

Good sources of omega-6s include nuts like walnuts, Brazil nuts, and seeds like sunflower and sesame. Good oils to choose include safflower and sunflower oils.

Myth #5-TAKING THE LATEST "WEIGHT LOSS PILL" WILL HELP YOU LOSE WEIGHT.

Where the myth may have come from. Appetite suppressants were placed on the market many many years ago. There are several different kinds of pills claiming to help you in the battle of the bulge. The reason you lose weight on these pills is because you are dieting and lowering your caloric intake. Again, going back to the reality of input vs. output. Some weight loss pills curb your appetite, some expand in your stomach making you feel full, and others help limit the absorption of your food. But as surely as you can find a pill to fit your needs on the road to weight loss, you can find a class-action lawsuit that is seeking damages for the bad those pills cause. Look it up, search it. You'll see the "reality" of the fantasy weight loss pill.

Body Check-Many of the weight loss supplements on the market today can do more harm than good. The ingredients in the pills are not regulated by the Food and Drug Administration. In other words, you can have more vitamin A than the label lists, or more caffeine, etc. The weight loss pill your friend or neighbor swears by wasn't even required to be tested by the FDA before it hit the market. The prescription drug industry has stringent protocols it must follow before a pill is released on the market.

This is not the case with dietary supplements... check it out- "FDA regulates both finished dietary supplement products and dietary ingredients under a different set of regulations than those covering "conventional" foods and drug products (prescription and Over-the-Counter). Under the Dietary Supplement Health and Education Act of 1994 (DSHEA), the dietary supplement or dietary ingredient manufacturer is responsible for ensuring that a dietary supplement or ingredient is safe before it is marketed. FDA is responsible for taking action against any unsafe dietary supplement product after it reaches the market. Generally, manufacturers do not need to register their products with FDA nor get FDA approval before producing or selling dietary supplements." Taken from www.fda.gov.

Smart Check-Stay clear of any weight loss supplements. Although these products can promise you the world and make you believe you can look like a model in three months time you will be disappointed. These drugs are unregulated by the FDA, so dangerous that lawsuits are constantly being filed in an attempt to recover damages that have been caused by these drugs, and they are potentially deadly to your nursing infant. Instead, opt for getting full by eating lots of vegetables and fiber, drinking plenty of water, and ingesting a steady supply of nutrients. Also, try natural appetite suppressants. I've listed several below. These can help curb your appetite and help you lower your caloric intake without the adverse side effects of popping a pill.

Natural weight loss appetite suppressants.

1. Handful of almonds-Almonds increase feelings of fullness and are also full of vitamin E, antioxidants, and magnesium.

2. Avocado-The fats founding avocados are heart-healthy monounsaturated fats. And they trick your body into a feeling of fullness. These fats send signals to your brain that tells your stomach that it's full.
3. Apples-One of the "superfoods" on this list, apples have pectin and soluble fiber that trigger a full feeling. Also, they regulate your glucose levels in the body and boost your energy levels. And because they require lots of chewing time they slow down your refrigerator and pantry raid.
4. Sweet Potatoes-Contains special starches that resist digestive enzymes and stays in your stomach longer making you feel full.
5. Vegetable Soup-Helps take the edge off your hunger.
6. Dark Chocolate (did someone say chocolate???)-Besides helping with sweet cravings, dark chocolate contains steric acid that slows digestion down and helps you feel fuller longer.
7. Green Tea-besides being a nice relaxing drink that staves off snacking, green tea actually has catechins in it that inhibits the movement of glucose into the cells, slows blood sugar, and prevents high insulin levels in the body.
8. Tofu-High in an isoflavone called genistein. This isoflavone has been shown to lower food intake by suppressing appetite.
9. Oatmeal-contains slow to digest carbohydrates that suppress the hunger hormone ghrelin
10. Green vegetables-high in fiber that will make you feel full for hours
11. Salmon-High in Omega-3 fatty acids. Fish high in Omega-3 increases the amount of the hormone leptin in your body and suppresses hunger.

12. Cinnamon-Helps lower your blood sugar levels to make you less hungry
13. Hot sauce-Sprinkle this on anything you can. Apparently for appetite suppression, the hotter the better. The spiciness keeps you from overeating.
14. Flax seeds-Sometimes you just gotta say "of course it's flax seeds." Flax seeds help you stay energized and help you feel full.
15. Salad-I probably eat at least two servings of salad everyday. It helps me feel full and keeps my calorie count down. Studies have shown that just a cup of salad eaten before your meal can signal your brain that you're full. It takes 20 minutes after you begin eating for the brain to recognize you are full and communicate this with your stomach. So eating that small salad before you eat your main course can help reduce the amount and calorie count of your meal.

Myth #6-WEGIHT LOSS SURGERY IS THE ONLY SOLUTION I HAVE TO LOSING WEIGHT.
This is just God-awful. And I'm going to get real frank with you. I've known lots of people who have had the surgery. I've seen countless commercials on television advertising gastric bypass or lap-band surgery as the only option for the obese. I've read several articles praising these procedures as saving people's lives. Even Medicaid (that's right, your tax dollars) will pay for this procedure. It's horrible. I've known people who have died after weight loss surgery.

Some have ended up in the critical care unit fighting for their lives. I've known others who will have a lifetime of stomach problems. It is not good to mess with your digestive tract. Do not do it. You will not live a pain-free life. You will always have problems with your digestion, and you might die. Instead, take the money you were going to spend on the surgery and invest in a long-term personal trainer who will work with you weekly to help you lose weight and get your diet under control. Giving tens of thousands of dollars to a surgeon and having him/her cut away part of your digestive system is BAD.

Body Check-This is a no-brainer. Do not do it. Don't you think you can get your hunger under control without cutting your body open and changing the way that God made you? Do you think you are that different than anyone else? Why can't you get your diet under control? And what kind of message does this surgery send to your children? Remember, kids follow in your footsteps, whether those are good or bad. Don't do it. 1% of surgery patients die, 20% of surgery patients need additional procedures (umm that's 1 out of 5 patients), and 1/3 of all patients develop a malnutrition disorder like osteoporosis or severe anemia as a result of their surgery because they can't absorb nutrients as they have reduced the area of the digestive tract that absorbs crucial vitamins and minerals. AND here's a bonus-when we age we ALLLLLL lose 30% of our bone mass. ALL OF US. So if you are a little on the thick side, your chances of developing osteoporosis are slim. If you are thin, your chances increase significantly. If you are thin because of weight loss surgery...you can count on getting the condition. Look at the BIG picture and stay away from weight loss surgery. It's not worth dying to be thin...

Smart Check-reduce the size of your stomach naturally by avoiding overeating, eating smaller more frequent meals, and getting plenty of water. Your stomach expands and reduces based on the amount of food you give it. You can train yourself to eat smaller meals and stop overeating. Choose high-fiber low-fat foods, and always opt for the lowest calorie snack. Read food labels, educate yourself on what you are eating and change your habits.

There is an abundance of scientific evidence out that points to obesity and excessive body fat being problems that begin in the blood brain barrier of the brain. This blood brain barrier is essentially like a gatekeeper, choosing what chemicals can enter the brain and affect the centers within. The diet program included in this guide has assumed that there is some truth to these scientific studies. It wouldn't be conducive to explain the specifics of these studies as it has taken many years in college for me to understand the biology of the body. There are also some scientific studies that link obesity to hormones. All of these have been taken into consideration and the diet plan for *Feed, Burp, Change, Repeat* resulted in the best possible eating plan with information taken from the latest research studies for both hypothesis. If you would like to check out these studies for yourself, search on the Internet for studies involving obesity and hormones or studies involving obesity and the brain.

I personally have had to look deeper into the subject of obesity and its effect on the brain and other body systems because of my own struggles with weight loss. As a science major I hold a special concentration of expertise in exercise and sports science and know a lot about weight loss and body fat reduction. I understand that you must eat less than you burn off in order to lose body fat. I also know how to calculate energy expenditure and I know how to eat for weight loss. Yet with my expertise and my background, I have had a huge struggle in this area. And for me it isn't just changing the amount of food I eat and the length of my exercise sessions that helps me to shed off unwanted pounds, I actually need to change what I eat and the timing of my meals. The diet Belinda designed for you is only a guide, a suggestion for you to lose your pregnancy weight. If you have a better diet that works for you, by all means use it! But if you choose to follow Belinda's plan, please understand that you must check with your doctor first and make sure you are able to begin a weight loss program…especially if you are nursing for two.

SURVIVING THE DIET

Diet. I always hated that word. Take out the T and you have the word DIE. But diet is easier to say than "food program" so I will refer to it as diet in the following section.

It seems like almost from birth I was always on some sort of diet. Really. Okay, well that may be a SLIGHT exaggeration but I have always struggled with my weight. I cannot eat foods high in sugar and fats. Just can't do it. Those foods always show up in the form of body fat after I eat them. Instantly. It seems like instantly anyways.

I remember being very young and not understanding why I couldn't eat like everyone else. I tried to blame my mom because she never was able to nurse me and statistically non-nursed babies are fatter children. I blamed my "fat set-point", when your body fat loses beyond this point your brain directs all sorts of fat reducing processes within the body to slow down to avoid any additional weight loss. I blamed the commercials that played on the television and relentlessly triggered my hunger. I blamed the stores for making healthier food much more expensive. I blamed the fast food chains for creating the dollar menus and two stations drive thru lanes that made it easier than ever to eat like crap. I always carried extra weight around with me. I ran, I rode my bike many many miles, I lifted heavy weights, and I dieted all the time. This was the lifestyle I had to maintain to fight the battle of the bulge. I never understood why I had to carry this cross in my life, but I've had to my whole life.

But out of some of the greatest trials in life, we are able to produce magnificent things, aren't we? Your weight loss journey is exactly that…a journey. You will be on this road for a while and you may have to make lifestyle changes for the rest of your days on this earth. But that's okay. Listen to your body and set your mind to be successful in this area. You will lose that twin belly and you will be back to normal weight soon enough. Just follow this diet as a guide and apply some variations, as they are needed to suit your lifestyle. Obviously if you can't cook a five course all organic meal, don't. Cook something easier but keep it healthy. Don't skip meals and grab a bag of chips to snack on. Don't grab the ice cream and eat it right out of the container. Do what makes sense. You can't outrun your fork…no matter how fast you run. So eat smart and have fun losing weight.

Before you begin the diet, you need to do some clean up around the house. No, not dusting or vacuuming, this clean up involves your fridge, freezer, and pantry. It's time to take an inventory of your food supplies and get rid of the bad food that dieters tend to grab when they are hungry. I've listed several foods that you might consider ditching. What do you do with them? Donate them to a food pantry, give them to a neighbor, or throw them out. It is not worth keeping them to avoid wasting food. There is no nutritional value in processed snack foods like chips, sugary foods, and soda. These are referred to as junk food for exactly that reason...they are junk.

Pantry:

Chips. These include pretzels and vegetable chips, and even natural chips. All of these are cooked in some sort of oil and contain salt. These are quick pleasure foods and will be the first thing you grab when you are hungry and you don't have time to make your food. Replace chips with quick to grab fruits and vegetables. I like to have baby carrots handy to munch on. It satisfies my hunger and my desire to chew.

Nuts. Peanuts, pistachios, walnuts, etc. Get rid of the nuts. These are high calorie foods and average 200-300 calories and 20 grams of fat for just a handful. Replace nuts with celery stalks. These are quite chewy and will satisfy your appetite to munch. In the diet there is a meal that contains almonds. I suggest getting those, dividing them up into baggies, and labeling the baggies with the days of the week. You will be less tempted to eat your week's supply of almonds if you remind yourself that those are taken ☺.

Sweets. Get rid of all sweets. Cookies, cakes, candies…all of it. Replace these with grapes. Grab grapes if your sweet tooth is calling you to eat sugar. Put grapes in baggies and portion out a serving so you don't mindlessly eat a bunch. Grab the grapes, step away from the kitchen, and satisfy your sweet tooth.

Peanut butter. As much as everyone thinks peanut butter is a protein…they are wrong. Peanut butter is a fat. With an average of 8 grams of fat and only 4-5 grams of protein per serving, and taking into account that fat nets over twice as many calories as protein, peanut butter is on average 70% fat! That's right 70% fat!! It's like taking oil and adding a small amount of whey protein powder to it and drinking it down. YUCK. Sure it tastes good but peanut butter is not very good for you. So ditch the jar. The kids don't need it anyways. Buy the peanut butter with the lowest possible fat per serving and purchase the all-natural kind to eat for your snack in the diet that's included. It's yucky so the kids won't want it anyways.

Sugary white bread. I know the kids need the bread for their snacks and lunches. So now you have to get creative. How are you going to ditch the white bread and replace it with whole wheat bread? Slowly…very slowly. Start with a gentle type of wheat like a white wheat. Then go for a honey wheat bread. Once they are used to that you can purchase whole wheat and go from there. Whole wheat bread is so much better for you than white bread. But you might have to get your children warmed up to it. They are your greatest resistance in eating healthy. However, you are the parent and ultimately they must eat what you decide to provide for them. So be creative and ease them into wheat bread but do not back down.

I'm sure there are other things in your pantry that you could ditch. I've listed the biggest potential problems but I'm sure there are others. You must continue to keep these bad foods out. Remember that you are in this for the long haul. Losing weight is not just about looking better it's about being better. Losing weight will help you live longer and healthier.

Now, for the next two weeks, you are going to help your body prepare to lose all the extra body fat you gained while pregnant. So your next assignment is to go to the closet and do an inventory of the sizes in there. Not the maternity clothes but the regular clothes. Don't fixate on your size 5 or 7 or whatever size you were pre-pregnancy. No, you want to figure out what size in there is about 10 pounds away from fitting. Grab that item of clothing and set it aside. We will deal with it later but for now trust me. Go get that pair of shorts or jeans or dress. And put it in a safe place.

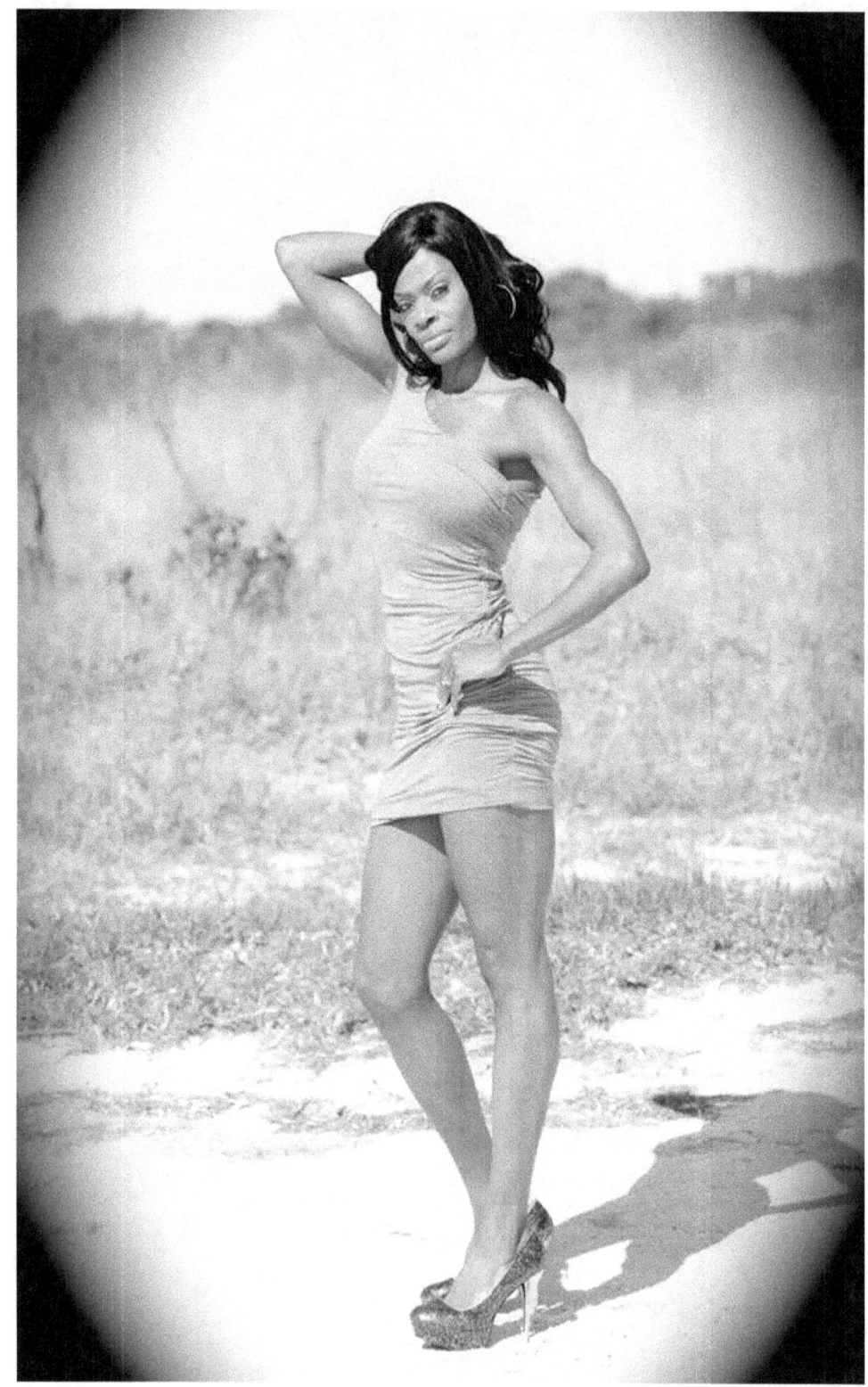

BODY BY BELINDA

This section was written by the only person I consider an expert in meal planning; my good friend and IFBB professional fitness competitor, Belinda Ann Hope. She has extensive experience in writing food programs for weight loss. Her own story of rising to the top in a brutal business where crash dieting is almost as common as breathing, is incredible. She struggled with being overweight. She has family members that struggle or have struggled with being overweight. You see this rock solid beauty is not naturally blessed to walk around with 8% body fat. She is naturally cursed to be fat. And Belinda is the perfect person to help you lose all that extra weight…because she's been there and she knows how to do it. At 38 years young, she won the most difficult competition of her life to earn IFBB professional status. 38! So don't even think that you aren't young enough to lose the body fat. She is still going strong and quickly approaching her forties!

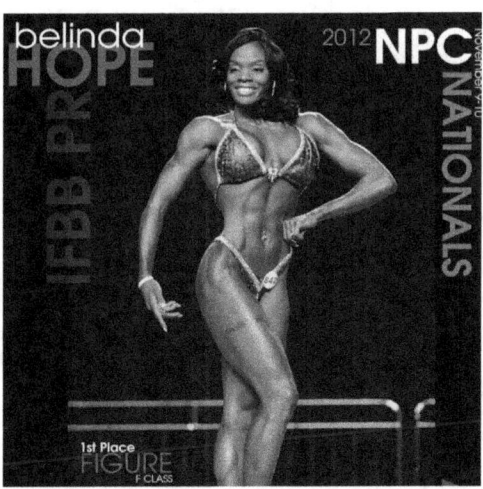

One day when I was talking to Belinda in the gym we worked at together, I asked her how long it took for her to recover from having her daughter. She smiled and blurted out "five years". I thought WHAT?? FIVE YEARS?? FOR HER? And I knew her dedication to lifting weights, eating right, and engaging in cardiovascular training was like none other I'd ever seen before. It wasn't uncommon to see Belinda training two to three times a day. And SHE took five years to recover from childbirth?? How long would it take me? How long is it going to take you?

How long depends on how much you are willing to do to lose weight. Your success is primarily linked to the diet. As much as you exercise to try and burn off body fat, if you don't get your diet under control, you will just be fighting a losing battle. It takes a deficit of 3500 calories to burn off just one pound of body fat. So this diet is crucial to your weight loss journey. It is a simple program that you can follow that won't leave you hungry. So sit back, relax, and enjoy. You are in good hands now…

Are you ready to get a "Body By Belinda"?

This meal program is only for those who are not nursing. As with any diet, please consult your physician to verify that you are ready to begin dieting. Also, if you are suffering from any complications from the childbirth (hypertension, injuries, etc.) you will want to check with your doctor. Recovering from childbirth is a long process. And ultimately it is TIME that will get your pre-pregnancy body back. So be patient. Rome wasn't built in a day. Your new body will take time to construct as well.

Meal 1 (breakfast)
3 hard boiled eggs (remove the yolk from two of the eggs)

1/2 cup cooked oatmeal OR
1 cup of brown rice OR
1 cup cream of wheat
10 almonds

(THIS NUTRITIONAL PLAN IS DESIGNED TO REMOVE PROCESSED FOODS BECAUSE THEY ARE LOADED WITH CHEMICALS THAT MAY ACTUALLY INHIBIT THE WEIGHT LOSS PROCESS) THEREFORE THE FIRST 2 WEEKS WILL INCLUDE NO PACKAGED FOODS LIKE CEREAL OR PROTEIN BARS

Meal 2 (BELINDA'S FAVORITE SNACK)
Small apple
1 tablespoon of natural peanut butter (level tablespoon NOT heaping ☺)

Meal 3
Chicken breast (3 or 4 oz)
1 cup of green beans
1 small sweet potato or small red potato

Meal 4
1/2 grapefruit
20 almonds

Meal 5
Lean protein (chicken, fish, sirloin, London broil)
Salad with oil and vinegar (try not to use packaged salad
dressing if you do look for dressing without msg or
chemicals of this nature) OR
2 cups green veggies like green beans or asparagus (this is
a natural diuretic)

After dinner snack if must have something
AIR POPPED POPCORN FROM KERNELS NOT THE
MICROWAVE STUFF OR
1 CUP OF GREEK YOGURT

With this diet program you will have plenty of meals that will
help you lose weight. How? It prevents hunger from setting
in and triggering the overeating that is so common with many
food programs. Getting a steady supply of food will help
stave off those cravings that send some people straight to the
pantry in a hunger fit. Also, the two "snack meals" meal 2
and 4, are quick grab snacks. You can prepare these ahead of
time and set them aside for the day until you are ready to eat
them. Since you are caring for two babies, time is always a
challenge. Eating right takes time. Do what you can to
prepare your day's food ahead of time just in case your day
becomes too challenging to stop and make food for yourself.
Skipping meals is NOT the best way to lose that weight!

After two weeks on the diet, you can adjust the plan to eat
things that appeal to your particular tastes. Here is what you
want to follow after two weeks

Meal 1 (breakfast)
3 hard boiled eggs (remove the yolk from two of the eggs)
OR

Scrambled eggs whites prepared with non-stick spray OR
1 Cup Low-fat (2% or 1%) cottage cheese OR
1 Cup of Greek Yogurt
2 slices of whole wheat toast plain or with small amount of light Smart Balance spread OR
1 Serving of High Fiber Cereal
1/2 cup cooked oatmeal OR
1 cup of brown rice OR
1 cup cream of wheat
10 almonds

Meal 2
1 Serving of fruit
1 tablespoon of natural peanut butter (level tablespoon NOT heaping ☺) OR
Mozzarella cheese stick

Meal 3
Lean protein (chicken, fish, sirloin, London broil 3 or 4 oz)
1 cup of green beans or small salad
1 small sweet potato or small red potato OR serving of brown rice

Meal 4
1 Serving of Fruit
20 almonds

Meal 5
Lean protein (chicken, fish, sirloin, London broil)
Salad with oil and vinegar OR
2 cups green veggies like green beans, broccoli, or asparagus

After dinner snack if must have something
AIR POPPED POPCORN FROM KERNELS NOT THE
MICROWAVE STUFF OR
1 CUP OF GREEK YOGURT

*For one of the above meals you can supplement with a protein shake but make sure it's pure protein without any added sweeteners and not a lot of ingredients (purchase this at the health food store) and mix it with 8 oz. skim milk.

As you can see, the diet doesn't change much. It is a simple plan that is easy to follow.

HOW TO STICK TO THE DIET

Now, the diet is good and makes sense to follow yet the reality is that monitoring everything that goes into your mouth is a challenge in itself.

I am the diet guinea pig. I know what to do and what not to do. 'Bad eating habits' is my middle name...well, not really it's Lynn. But I do have a lot of experience in this area. I had to change every eating habit I've had at one point or another in my life. I've compiled some tips below to help you keep on track to losing all that baby weight!

1. Water. Drink plenty of water throughout the day to help stave off hunger and help you eat less at meals. However, too much water at one sitting can actually stretch your stomach out so sip all day for the best results.
2. Fiber. Choose high-fiber foods when picking your meals. This includes fruits with at least 5 grams of fiber per serving (apples are awesome and filled with fiber), whole grains, vegetables, and beans. You need between 25-30 grams of fiber every day. They've studied dieters and

found that the dieters who kept a high-fiber diet after they lost their weight managed to keep the weight off and didn't gain it back while the low fiber dieters rebounded and gained a good portion of their weight back.

3. Stay away from sugar and refined foods. Choose the foods that have the LEAST amount of ingredients on the back of the box.

4. Avoid eating anything with MSG. That's monosodium glutamate. It's like cyanide for your body. Many salad dressings, especially creamy ones, have this. Look on the nutrition label around the middle of the list0that's usually where they hide it ☺.

5. Avoid animal fat. Choose lean cuts of beef, chicken, and fish. Animal fat is FULL of saturated fat. Saturated fat is an inflammatory agent on the body as well as an amplifier of cholesterol levels. Don't eat the skin on poultry. Don't choose the steak with the fat in it, and go for non-fat or low-fat dairy products.

6. Don't eat trans fats. These are the hydrogenated vegetable oils used in most processed food and fast foods. Trans fats are so bad for you that some cities want to ban the use of them in their restaurants entirely.

7. Keep portions moderate. If you must have a cookie and cheat, keep that cookie to half a cookie or one cookie. Throw the rest out.

8. Eat a variety of foods. Eating the same every day can get very boring and it isn't as healthy for you as varying your diet.

9. Stay away from alcohol. If you must have a drink, keep it to one and only have it once in a while. Alcohol is like eating straight sugar for your body. It adds an abundance of calories to your diet without supplying you with any nutrients. Stay away from it. If you can't, use it as a pound reward. For every 5 lbs you lose, reward yourself with a drink. But only if you can't seem to let it go entirely. I haven't had a drop of alcohol in over 6 years. And I really don't miss it at all. Plus I know I'm sending a

great message to my kids. How can I convince them to stay away from drinking when I'm doing it myself??

CHAPTER EIGHT
A healthy everlasting marriage (or partnership) caring for twins

This section I almost couldn't write. Seriously. My husband and I had PROBLEMS. Major ones. He worked extra hours to bring in more money for our expanding family, I was at home pouring my heart and life into the children, and we let our marriage slip further and further away. Some days we were so in love it made our boys groan and run the other way, but other days we it seemed we disagreed about everything and were ready to walk out on each other (my husband actually DID walk out when the twins were three weeks old-for about two hours). How can the super blessing of twins cause two people who committed to spend the rest of their lives together to want to give up and walk away from their marriage?

If you are experiencing marriage issues, you are not alone. As much enjoyment as your new bundles bring, they also bring lots of issues to the table. There is a definite financial strain. There is a time strain. There is extra stress in the household. Fears and doubts can creep in. Your heart gets pulled away from each other as you literally give everything you've got to taking care of two babies. You may feel depressed and anxious especially as your hormone levels return to 'normal'. He may feel overwhelmed with the financial burden of taking care of the larger family (or vice versa).

So what is the solution? What can you do to keep your marriage together? How can you survive the next 18+ years??? You must take time out and invest in your marriage. That is the great key to a long happy marriage. Investment. And it starts right here.

A healthy marriage

First let's discuss what we all want to achieve for our marriages-a healthy marriage. A healthy marriage, what does it look like? Do you agree on everything? Do you both enjoy each other's company all the time? Are you both able to enjoy satisfying sex and are both mutually in agreement about how often that occurs?

Ummm.. NOT. A healthy marriage is an ever changing and developing process that takes time, lots of time, to develop. A healthy marriage will endure through the ups and downs and will get stronger as the years go on. Perfection will never be achieved because you are two different people. However, over time eventually you will understand the other person's position on many things and will be able to grow together to mutually respect each another for your unique and very different opinions. Sex will also go up and down. Literally. Sometimes you may hit a slam-dunk in the bedroom, both of you ending a hot lovemaking session completely exhausted yet satisfied. Other times one of you may have an awesome night but leave the other person feeling left out. And one of the worst moments, which my husband and I have had several, when neither one of you finishes the session and you stop midway through to turn over and go to bed. One thing you can be sure of-sex is always different. And your level of satisfaction is different too.

So let's talk about sex first...

Successful sex

Sex can be successful. Early on in your marriage, sex was incredible. It was easy to find the time to make love, and both of you were often so in tuned to each other that the rest of the world didn't matter. The house could be on fire and you probably wouldn't even notice. It was all and I mean ALL about the two of you. But then the pregnancy happened. And sex probably hit an all time high. With extra hormones comes extra passion for the woman. Life couldn't get better could it? Then the babies come, you have six weeks off, and lovemaking commences. And it's hotter than ever. Well, for a few months. Then the stress of the babies, the money stress, the time stress…all come into a big reality check for the both of you. What used to be easy seems more like a job. What can you do?

Begin by understanding why the two of you now have big differences in what you want and how you want it. Sex is a mind thing for the woman and a body thing for the man. Although there are some men that use their emotions more during intimacy and there are some women who are more physically involved, most often this is the case in every marriage. Women cannot compartmentalize their day. In other words, women stay home all day with the kids and literally their day goes to bed with them in their mind. Men, on the other hand, can have the worst day ever and still go to bed ready to engage in sex. Women are totally connected with everything while men separate everything. This is the main reason why women and men generally do not share the same passion for intercourse.

So if you don't share the same passion, don't worry. It does not mean that you aren't meant for each other. It simply means that you are different. And different is precisely how you were designed. So first thing's first, you must get on the same page when it comes to sex. This means a little extra work for the woman and extra work for the man as well.

For the women out there…in case you hadn't noticed before, men are visual when it comes to intimacy. They'd rather have the lights on brightly and you in lingerie that will soon be ripped from your body. You in your post-pregnancy shape probably want the room pitch black, and prefer wearing an outfit that thoroughly covers you. Meet your husband halfway here. Opt for dimming the lights or lighting candles to give the room a soft yet flattering glow. Go out to the mall and buy some pretty pieces of lingerie that cover you yet keep you looking much sexier than the drape you wore while pregnant. That is about all you need to do for him. And by all means, you will probably need to have sex more often than you want to. He has a much higher sex drive (well, in most marriages). Just try to relax and meet his needs as much as you can. But when pain sets in or you aren't feeling very good, do something else to finish the night. The last thing he wants to do is hurt you.

For the men out there…you must meet your wife in her world and engage in conversation and non-sexual touching before you enter the bedroom. The worst thing you can do to your wife is come home from work, get busy with the computer, the kids, the things that need fixing around the house…and completely ignore her needs. Then travel to bed and expect her to be ready. This is probably one of the biggest mistakes men make. Your woman needs to separate from her day. And you are the one who needs to help her do that. If you don't, she will take her entire day to bed with you. And you will not be the only thing on her mind as you are engaging in foreplay. So avoid the competition with her day and spend some quality time sitting next to her on the couch, help her with the chores and the children, and connect with her in her world.

Sex is no longer about you; it's all about your spouse. Make it all about your spouse and your spouse will return the favor. Then sex will be amazing. Just trust me on this one. Sex was an area where we struggled a lot after the twins were born.

Next, make sure when the two of you are together, that you communicate how you feel. I still have issues with my stomach and it's been 2 years since I had the twins. Some nights my stomach hurts so bad I want to cry. Obviously on this night we would need to work around my stomach. The only way my husband knows I am in pain is if I tell him. Also, some nights I need extra TLC before we take our clothes off. This is again something I need to communicate to my partner. We've tried the whole mind reading thing but apparently men aren't mind readers…so you must stick to telling him everything you can to make the bedroom experience more pleasurable for the two of you.

Don't ditch the foreplay. The both of you have been given something so special. Sex is the covenant seal for your marriage. You are supposed to enjoy it, and find pleasure in it. But lately you may be feeling rushed to fit it into your schedule. Often I used to wear myself out by the time kids were put to bed and it was our turn for time together. I would fall asleep before my husband would have a chance to start anything. Or if we started, I'd get so tired I would fight falling asleep. This is not the best way to have a sex life. And this is where foreplay is critical to success. Foreplay keeps both of you engaged in the moment. Foreplay draws you into each other and helps you to focus. Foreplay heightens your senses and keeps you alert for sex. Foreplay is an important aspect of a successful sex life.

Communicate. And now you go back to communication.
Foreplay is done successfully if both of you have a clear
understanding of what turns your spouse on. So take some
time out with each other, explore each other's bodies, and
discover the great spots and the best methods you can use to
have successful foreplay. This is going to take a little work,
and chances are some spots may have changed particularly for
the woman post-baby. No worries. Just start at the head and
work your way down.

Slow down. Vary your speed and intensity while lovemaking.
You aren't running a sprint race. Marriage is more of a
marathon. So while you are engaging in lovemaking, take it
slow, pay attention to each other's bodies, and enjoy. Slow
down and speed up…and then slow back down again. Take
time with each other. You both spent all day making time for
everyone else, kids, work, family, and friends. Now it's time
to devote your attention to each other.

Make it about your spouse. Do it for the other person. Wives,
make love for your husband's pleasure. Husbands, make love
for your wife's pleasure. Don't do it for yourselves, do it for
each other. This automatically tunes you into your partner's
needs and will make sex more satisfying for both of you.

Experiment. Talk about what your desires are, even if they
are a little out of the ordinary for your regular sex life.
Explore options for sex that you are both comfortable with,
and utilize those methods. This may be different positions,
different accessories like clothing or creams, or different
places to make love at. Agree that unless it is mutually agreed
upon, that you will not do it. Your comfort level and
confidence is key to successful experimentation.

Time it. Lovemaking may not be the best at night any more.
With the new babies and new demands that creep into your
marriage, you might have to time your sessions differently.
For the first several months our lovemaking sessions had to be
done during the day. Because by nightfall I was totally spent
and we would just fall asleep together in the middle of
foreplay. So we stole moments when we could steal them,
and made sure no one would catch us.

Schedule it. If your schedule is tight, try scheduling your
sessions. Discuss with your partner times and days that
lovemaking can be scheduled in. I know, this sounds real
boring but it's not. If you know it is your lovemaking night,
you can prepare the children for bed and take a nice warm
bath to get cleaned up and in the mood. And if you know it's
not a night then you can ditch the bath and get into cleaning
the house or relaxing to a movie or book…whatever you need
to do. Scheduling in sex doesn't make your marriage boring,
it makes is less chaotic as the uncertainty of what the night
will bring the two of you is solved.

The 'Date Night' dilemma.

This was a dilemma my husband and I struggled with a lot
when we were new parents of twins. Date nights seemed
impossible. Yet all the marriage experts will tell you the same
thing "go out once a week on a date night." Yeah, right. How
are we supposed to do that when we are broke and no one in
their right mind will watch ALL these kids anyways (we have
5 at home who need to be watched)? What are you to do
when the only possible solution seems virtually impossible for
you TO do? It's the perfect dilemma for a little creativity.

My husband and I had to approach the date night thing differently. We found when we went out together we would have to keep our date short. The long 4 or 5 hour dates had to be a thing of the past, at least for a little while. We opted to go and walk on the beach or share an ice cream rather than go out to dinner and a movie. Date night does not need to be very long. Just take time out together outside of your home, even if it's only for a quick hour. Something is always better than nothing.

Keep your date nights cheap. Unless you are one of the lucky ones with an ample supply of money, chances are you have been spending your date money on an endless supply of diapers. If you go out to dinner and spend money you might simply run out of diapers by the end of the month (my husband and I did this!). So when you go out together, keep the dates nice and inexpensive. Here are some great suggestions to help reignite that lost flame at a low price…

Go for a walk to an ice cream shop. If the weather doesn't allow a walk, hop in the car and drive there but take the long way. The time you spend traveling to the shop is a great opportunity to talk through some things. And when you arrive to your destination, quit talking serious and allow small talk on your date. For my husband and I we really have a lot of important stuff to talk about and we find that sometimes we have to cut the conversation off and allow light small talk to fill our time together. If we don't do this then we will never stop talking about the children.

Go for a drive in the car to see the sunset on the beach or lake. Grab extra blankets so you can get out of the car and sit on the ground. Or if you stay in the car, use those blankets to cover up and cuddle together. You let the night dictate where your passion goes. Just be smart and enjoy!

Rent a movie and watch it together (kids will need to be watched at someone else's home). Pick a romantic movie or an action movie with a hot steamy couple in it. Most husbands get turned on by seeing sex scenes in movies. But make sure you choose a flick that won't have you feeling less sexy because of the actress in it. I will pick a movie with my favorite actress and I will usually research the film so I can be prepared for those naked parts. I'm still mourning my size 5 body and until I get back there I tend to feel very self-conscious about myself. Some movies can literally send me crying to my room. So choose wisely and for God's sake DO NOT LET YOUR HUSBAND PICK THE MOVIE ☺.

Both of you cook your favorite meal together and sit down for a romantic candlelight dinner with soft music playing in background (kids will need to be watched at someone else's home). Pick romantic dishes that you can share feeding each other with. Choose items like strawberries dipped in chocolate, or steak that you can feed to each other. Any dish can be romantic if it tastes good. So be creative and plan ahead.

Go 'park' somewhere and talk for a bit. Be prepared for other things to happen…I usually wore a skirt on our 'park' dates. We got very hot and heavy in the car on our third date after the twins. I think that night for my husband it was four times. Twice in the car and twice when we got back home. One of man's greatest needs is sex. So don't worry about feeling a little raunchy. You are married and you are supposed to enjoy each other.

Drive to a new town and go to a coffee shop and sit for a while. This is nice because no one knows you and you can really relax and spend time talking together the whole drive out there. Sometimes the best thing the two of you can do is just go away for a bit. Kind of like a mini escape. Don't worry the kids are fine. Just plan the time out so you won't be late arriving back home.

Go out to dinner but share a meal. Or use a coupon to make it less expensive. My husband and I had a buy one get one free coupon for an entrée at a restaurant we had never been to before. We used it and had a very nice time out together and the total bill was $15.00!

Make sure you take advantage of any company dinners or outings. I know this sounds boring but you will have a great time ditching the dinner after you eat and walking off on your own. At my husband's Christmas party we ate and made our exit quickly afterwards. We had a delightful time walking around the area outside the banquet hall and then sat in the car and talked.

Plan a his and hers massage session at home (again kids need to be at someone else's house). Get some good massage oil and take turns massaging each other. It will help you relax together and will also be great foreplay for a romantic night together. I suggest wearing something sexy to help set the mood. And don't forget to drag food and drink to your room so you can easily snack afterwards.

Go to the park and find a wonderful bench with a great view to talk the night away. Bring a picnic meal and dine together. I suggest bringing gum to freshen up afterwards and bring a few blankets in case you end up laying on the ground or running to the car and want to cover up ☺.

Go for a romantic bike ride and plan on stopping for a coffee, drink, or an ice cream along the way. This is great because you can talk all the way to the shop and once you arrive at your destination you can both relax together and rekindle romance. An added bonus for the woman is that you've burned calories on the way there and on the way back, making you fell a little less guilty about devouring that double scoop ice cream cone.

Go to the local driving range or mini golf course. Wager something sexual to the winner. It will definitely make the time playful. Men love competition and sports. And to do the two together while throwing in a sexual undertone to the night is a formula for total turn on for him.

Go hiking together. Search on the Internet for great hiking trails near you. Bring something to drink and a blanket just in case you want to stop along the way. And women, I suggest wearing something he loves on you like short shorts or an easy accessible skirt so you can get his heart racing and rekindle some great romance.

Go stargazing together at your favorite outdoor spot. Today you don't even need a telescope and a chart to do this. My husband uses an app on his phone and he points it towards the sky to find all the constellations. It is fun and very romantic. Every time you find a system, agree to give each other a kiss.

Of course you can't always get a baby sitter. Some nights there may not be enough time. Some weeks you simply don't have the cash. And if a child is feeling ill there is no way you will be able to go. AHA. This is time for relationship rescue. And don't worry, even the best marriages need extra work to be successful. I've included here a list of things you can do without involving the cost of a babysitter. My suggestion is to plan 'free date nights' at least once a week. Use these nights in addition to date nights. It's kind of like the back up plan for the two of you. And trust me you will need a back up plan with twins!

FREE DATE NIGHT IDEAS AT HOME

Rent a movie and plan on putting the kids to bed early. Watch the movie in your room, light a candle, and cuddle in bed together. Let things happen naturally. Couples need time and touch every single day. This is a great way to rekindle lost romance.

Get up early before the kids rise and eat breakfast together. Instead of hopping on the computer or reading the newspaper, put all distractions away and focus on each other. Plan to eat something that doesn't make too much noise to cook. Or pick up bagels and cream cheese from the local bakery and enjoy someone else doing the cooking for you!

Go outside and pitch a tent in the backyard. After you put the babies to bed venture outdoors for a romantic fire and some much needed alone time. Take advantage of the time together and when you are finished rekindling the romance, put the fire out and head back inside to the bedroom.

Take a shower together by candlelight. You will probably not get very clean during this shower but no worries. It isn't a shower for that. My husband and I love to take a hot steamy shower together and have a little foreplay action in the shower. Then we would change our location to the bedroom to finish what we had started.

Put the kids to bed early and have a romantic candlelight dinner together. Your twins should go to sleep around 8p.m. or 8:30p.m. every night. If that is too late for the two of you, wake them up earlier from their late nap. Chances are they will fall asleep early for the night and you can have a few hours to yourselves before sleep takes over for the two of you.

After the twins are settled for the night, plan on eating ice cream on the front or back porch together and make it a date. You can get creative and set up a table and some chairs for your ice cream date. If you already have them set up outside throw a fun tablecloth over the table just to spice up the atmosphere.

Have a drink together. Set up an area either outside or in and enjoy a few drinks together by candlelight. Just like some of your first dates when you took time out and sipped beverages at the bar, escape mentally from your daily mom and dad duties and relax together. If you don't drink alcohol choose non-alcoholic beverages.

Share a dessert. As simple as this is, it works. Sharing a dessert like ice cream on top of brownies or a nice big slice of cake can be very romantic. And the messier the dessert is the better. Take turns wiping the hot fudge or frosting from each other's mouths. Deserts can be so much fun.

Grab your favorite blanket and head to the fire. Set up a romantic fire in the fireplace and plan to camp out in front for a while. Some soft music playing in the background will help set the mood.

Get under the covers and watch a movie in the living room. Wear something super comfortable and easily accessible. Touching each other during the movie is a great way to enjoy foreplay. And the added bonus is that you get to snuggle together for hours while the movie plays. Make sure your snacks and drinks are on the table next to you so neither one of you has to get up and break the connection. Also make sure you use the bathroom ahead of time.

Grab a blanket and sit down in front of the television with a picnic dinner. It may seem silly to do since the dining table is literally in the next room but it is a way to switch things up. Choose food you can feed to each other.

Have a theme night. You should dress, eat dinner, and watch a movie all related to your chosen theme. IF you go western, dress like a cowgirl and cowboy, cook some bar-b-que, and watch a western movie. Would you rather go French? Choose a black and white top, make some delicious French entrees and serve it with a side of French onion soup, and watch a sexy French movie.

Play a game. Yes, this will do wonders for your relationship. Either break out the board games or hook up the video games. Take time out and focus on having a great time, just the two of you.

Dance the night away. Get dressed up and throw in some of your favorite songs to dance to. Make sure you choose some slow songs to add to the mix. And just make room for your own private dance floor. Lighting candles around the room will add to the sexiness of the evening.

Work out together. Set up a fun weight training area in the garage or another room and create a fun workout circuit to do together. Things will get heated as you workout so after you are done working out, make a mad dash to the shower and take a shower together. Finish this night off in the bedroom. Just make sure you don't wake the kids.

GETTING RID OF THE NEGATIVES

Now that you've been working on the time thing with your partner, it's time to venture into some of the negative things that can affect your relationship. Even when dates and romance are going well, negativity can come in and destroy some of the best marriages. The biggest negative item to deal with is definitely fear. Fear is a relationship killer!

Often times it creeps up without any warning. There are many causes of fear, but one of the biggest causes is past relationship failure.

So let's go over ways you can get rid of fear. Before it enters into your relationship and destroys.

First deal with the past issues. This means talking talking and more talking.

Second, stop doing things to trigger fear in each other.

Ways to trigger fear in women...

1. Boss her around by telling her what to do.
2. Being short with her.
3. Neglecting her by ignoring her.
4. Ignore her feelings.
5. Giving the cold shoulder.
6. Take her for granted.

7. Limit her spending critically instead of deciding on financial issues together.
8. Tell her to stop worrying, to get over it, and tell her she's making a big deal out of nothing.
9. Letting her know that she talks too much.
10. Saying anything negative about her weight.
11. Pout.
12. Shut down or totally withdraw.
13. Threaten to quit your job.
14. Become flirty with other women. Even friend's wives or "taken" women.
15. Look at other women for more than a glance. Even on the television this can trigger a long battle for the two of you.
16. Tell her she's just like her mom.
17. Complain to her about her girlfriends.
18. Don't listen to her ideas.
19. Buy a sports car/motorcycle for yourself.

Ways to trigger fear in a man…

1. Correct what he says.
2. Question his judgment or lack or judgment.
3. Don't include him and consult him in important decisions.
4. Keep him from doing things to help you out.
5. Make him feel inadequate.
6. Overreact, yes even on PMS days you must try to stay calm around him.
7. Ignore what his desires are.
8. Focus and complain about what you don't have or didn't get.
9. Withhold praise from him.
10. Speak to him using a harsh tone.
11. Be spontaneous and spring things on him abruptly (unless it's a surprise date).
12. Undermine his authority, especially in front of the kids.

13. Use condescending tones.
14. Criticize his personality.
15. Complain about his job.
16. Show little interest in what he is interested in.
17. Criticize his family no matter how crazy they are.
18. Make comparisons to other men, especially exes.
19. Focus on your state of unhappiness.
20. Value friends before him. Put friends first.

When my husband and I sat down and put together this list, we realized we had been doing several of the items on it to each other. We printed out a copy of it and now review it together so that we have it in our memory. Our goal is to quit doing all things on the list to each other. You should print out a copy too. I've enclosed a sheet located at the end of the book for you to copy and print out so you can review it together too. It really helps.

Most couples don't realize how easily they can fall into this trap of triggering fear in their partner. Fear will kill any marriage. And it creeps in over time. It's like a bad habit and you must change your pattern of behavior to change the result. Even in cases of blatant verbal abuse, using fear to deliberately control your partner, this list can literally save your marriage by bringing the verbal abuse to an end. Just agree together that you will stop triggering fear in each other and move forward. You cannot change the past you can only change the present and direct change for your future.

Third, make a list of grievances. Sit down together and make two lists. The women need to make a list of things the men have done to cause hurt, and the men should do the same list for the women. Past hurts. Once you are finished, breathe, pray, do something to calm down. And then go over your lists together. Unresolved tension in your relationship will one day come to the surface and could cause major issues in your marriage. This list is for those tensions. As you go through the lists, don't judge each other or make your partner feel stupid for writing certain items down. This is their heart not yours. Just because you think it's ridiculous doesn't mean it hasn't caused major hurt in the other person's heart. Be sensitive and understanding with these lists.

Go line-by-line alternating lists, and allow open discussion of every item individually. There are items on the lists that neither one of you probably knew caused any issues. There are probably other items on the lists that both of you thought were resolved long ago. This is an important habit to continue long into your marriage. Often parents of twins run around so busy that there isn't much time, except in the beginning when the twins are newborn, to have discussions. These lists are a great resource to use over and over again.

When you feel the item has been properly resolved...through apology, hugging, explaining, praying, etc...then you can cross it off the list. Once you are through the list if there are any items that have not been crossed off, you should go to bed and attempt to address it the following day. Sometimes a little thinking and a little sleep will spark an idea that may help resolve that issue the very next day.

Fourth, talk about the things that cause you to fear in your everyday routines. This could be items like coming home late for work, not answering the cell phone at a certain hour, or relationships with the opposite sex that cause concern. Since the two of you are very different people, there will be items that each one of you are doing that cause unrest in your partner that you were not aware was causing a problem whatsoever. And it is probably fixable. So fix it ☺.

Fifth, put up relationship boundaries. I am going to list my marriage boundaries to give you an idea of what we had to do to protect our relationship.

1. Discuss what boundaries you need to have for travel with the opposite sex. We do not travel in a car alone with the opposite sex. This is a big one. If you have a job that requires the opposite sex to travel with you, either get another person to come along or call your spouse on the phone to inform him/her of what is happening.
2. Discuss what boundaries you need to have for social networking. We do not accept any single persons of the opposite sex on Facebook or other social networking sites

unless it is a mutually agreed upon friend or family member. If you are married, you should be friends with married couples. Period. Even on the Internet. Single people can DESTROY your marriage.

3. Address what is acceptable for sharing information and whom it is acceptable to share that information with. We do not share information about our relationship with the opposite sex. Even if it seems innocent, it is not. There are people out there that will try to hurt your marriage. Even the innocent looking young girl at the flower shop may be out to grab your husband as he harmlessly explains how he is going to purchase flowers and get romantic with you. Or the woman at the bakery shop, etc. Or the guy at the car shop...

4. Make movie boundaries. We do not watch movies with nudity. Period. If it contains nudity, unless it is very brief, we won't watch the film or we will skip quickly through the nude scenes. Figure out what is acceptable in your home. I personally don't think I should be drooling over a naked guy on the big screen, and my husband shouldn't be lusting after a naked woman. We should be doing that with each other. But that is our boundary. Maybe the two of you won't have such a strict movie boundary. Nothing is right or wrong. It is only right or wrong for YOUR marriage. So discuss this openly with your partner. And stick to that boundary.

Once you stop triggering fear in each other, and work to resolve past fears, you can enjoy a fear free relationship. It will take time but it is something that can be achieved and will help you enjoy a lifelong happy marriage.

Listen to each other

Okay, men. Quit rolling your eyes. I know for the majority of couples the woman talks WAY more than the man. But men, did you know that listening to your wife is the best way to get her in the mood for sex? Do I have your attention now?

Communication is key to a happy marriage. Unfortunately when the babies come out and into your world, finding the opportunity to communicate can be quite challenging, especially if one of the babies is a crier. But if you don't talk, how will you know each other's needs? Relationships are not built on ESP alone. You must get into the habit of having regular daily communication. And not just a "hi, what's for dinner" or "can you get me two bottles please?" The daily talks must have depth to them, contain some level of discussion, and solve some type of situation or issue.

Women you must open up to your husband. Your husband will most likely not take the initiative to begin a discussion. If you sit around the house all evening and wait for him to spark a talk, you will go to bed disappointed. So one of your jobs in the whole "better communication" gig is to corner your husband and be in charge of what time and where you will have your daily conversation. You will also need to help him be the communicator you want him to be. This means keeping him focused on the conversation by keeping your points short and giving him positive feedback when he has done a great job. Men want the EDITED version of what you are sharing. They respond better to shorter talks. Always keep that in mind, especially when you are discussing important issues. Don't talk forever because he will tune you out.

Men, I know it's tough to communicate. You would rather chill out and relax, watch television, fix something on your to do list, or surf the Internet. Having conversation isn't one of your preferred things to do. Your needs are quite different from hers in this area. But don't worry I have put together some tips that will help you on your road to better communication and a happier marriage.

SURVIVING THE TALKS

1. FOCUS. First things first, FOCUS. This is where you must shut off the television, the computer, your cell phone, and put away all potential distractions. Giving your wife your undivided attention is the first step on the road to better communication.
2. REPEAT. Repeat back to your wife key points of the discussion. This shows her that you are engaged in the talk. Show her you care about what she is saying and that you are really listening to her.
3. SHUT. Shut your mouth. Don't interrupt even if she seems like she's more of a marathon runner than a sprinter in the communication department. Your wife is trying to share her day with you so you can give her comfort. She is talking to YOU not her girlfriends. This is a special moment don't blow it.
4. DON'T SOLVE. Only solve the problem if it is something you should solve. Often women just want a shoulder to lean on not a counselor. Listen for the sake of listening to her needs. And solve or give advice only when she seems willing to receive it.
5. DON'T EVER BE A JERK. Don't make her feel she is wrong or belittle her. Don't ever tell her she has a stupid opinion. Your goal is to validate her feelings not make fun of them. Ignoring this step is a one-way ticket to sleeping the night on the couch. If you don't believe it, try this and see where you end up for the night.
6. DON'T HAVE THE LAST WORD. This is something I've seen over and over again with men and women. Men are so competitive by nature that they are adamant about having the last word in the conversations even if it is a stupid last word or phrase that they add. Don't do this. If she talks for longer (which will probably happen) don't insist on having the last word. She will most likely always win the battle of words

with you. So be satisfied with letting her end the conversation. It will make her feel so much better.

Men and women are very different in the way they think through issues and in the way they respond to problems. Women have a brain that switches from the right to left side during conversation. In other words, women can think about many items during the same conversation. A woman's brain is a queen multi-task machine, that's why it is so easy for women to do many things at once. During conversation one subject may lead to twelve in her mind. So women, be mindful of the temptation to spill out all your guts and discuss everything that comes to your mind in one conversation. Stick to one or two key points and leave the rest for another day.

Men's brains work more like a strong machine that does best performing one job at a time. Men compartmentalize everything. One thing does not lead to another in their brain. Their brains have stellar focus. So when men are engaged in conversation as long as they keep the distractions to a minimum, they are very good at solving one problem at a time. So men, realize that you may need to bend a little in this area and open your mind up to one subject turning into a few.

It is okay to disagree and even sometimes argue when you are talking. But always disagree in a fair and respectful manner and make sure that you both have equal opportunity to share your differences. Sometimes you might need to do more footwork to solve an issue, like consult your parents, pastor, or find books and articles relative to what you are battling. There is always a solution if you are willing to search for it.

Get romantic

What is romance? Oftentimes men and women have a very different idea of what romance is.

Historically men have fallen short in this. So instead of brushing up on their skills they essentially "give up". Which is the worst thing you can do for a woman. Women thrive on romance. If you work to bring romance into your daily relationship, your marriage will stand the test of time. Romance literally carries your bond through life's ups and downs. Romance is the glue that holds it all together.

Being romantic varies widely from person to person, but basically, romance involves doing something to express affection in a meaningful and unexpected way. A true act of romance requires some level of creativity and sincerity, and needs to be inspired by love. While feeling affection for someone might be fairly easy, translating it into romance or a romantic gesture usually is not. There are ideas for romance everywhere, located in books, movies, t.v. shows, the Internet, and other people, but true romance comes from within. True romance comes from the heart.

SURVIVING ROMANCE

I've put together some tips to help enhance your romantic experience. These are only suggestions so look them over and adapt the ideas that fit your specific needs. Romance is never a one size fits all. And romance can change as often as the days change. Pay attention to each other and communicate if your romantic needs are not being met. And have fun bringing that spark back into your marriage.

1. PERSONAL. Make it personal. Ditch the stereotypical roses and candles and think about what really gets your partner swept off his/her feet. Step into his/her world and meet in that realm. Recognize what makes your spouse different than you and go out of your way to make them feel special. What lights up your spouse's eyes? What makes him/her feel full of life? Is it talking? Walking? Watching a show or movie? Maybe it will take

nothing more than a dimly lit room and some cuddling. Romance is not in things. It's in people. So spend some time in your spouse's world and meet his/her unique needs.

2. COURT THEM. Why do you think that the spark is gone? Is it that the two of you are getting too comfortable with each other? Well, why don't you play a game of pretend? Pretend that you and your spouse have just met. What can you do to make him/her fall in love with you again? Maybe it's wearing that sexy dress or men maybe you need to keep close shaven. Maybe there was a favorite cologne or perfume...or maybe your spouse fell for you because you were spontaneous. Win your partner over again. Impress your spouse. Make him/her fall in love with you all over again.

3. DO SOMETHING SPONTANEOUS. You need to break the monotony of the relationship. Often times when people marry, everything gets old and predictable. Gone are the days when the anticipation of what your partner could do next would fill your thoughts. You've gotten so predictable. Same text messages, same phone calls, same time you see each other. Now every communication is filled with problem solving, every gesture is about the long haul rather than the moment. To be romantic, you must reintroduce the excitement that you once had at the beginning of the relationship. So do something different. Grab flowers and bring them to your wife. Women get the babies to bed early and grab your new piece of lingerie, put it on, and wait in bed. Meet your spouse at his/her work for lunch. Do something totally different, something that your partner would not expect. Even as I am writing this, I have decided to leave my computer and head upstairs to be in bed when my husband gets up. I am normally downstairs typing away ☺.

4. DETAILS. Focus on the small things. Romance was never meant to be expensive. As a matter of fact romance should typically be free. There are a million ways for you to make your partner feel loved and special. Meet them in

their world and do something nice for them. Take your regular dinner and light some nice candles. Men run a special bath for her and give her 30 minutes of peace to soak in the tub. You don't have to change your schedule to be romantic. Just add a little bit of extra in the middle of your normal routine.

5. GRATITUDE. Show that person how truly special they are by being grateful for their presence in your life. Continually remind your partner that he/she has made your life better. A few simple kind words will go a long way.

As I wrote this section about romance, I was falling short in my own marriage. And my husband was following suit. It had been at least 3 weeks since we'd made love, we were down to a hello and goodbye kiss daily, and we hadn't been out together or in together for weeks. He was working about 25 hours of overtime every paycheck, which meant I was working 25 hours overtime with the twins at home, and we had on average 2 football games to attend weekly with 2 boys in tackle football. There wasn't enough time in the day for us, for each other, and especially for romance. Our marriage was dying. It's amazing how two people can fall away so quickly when they have twins. I had heard about the divorce rate being much higher for parents of twins, but I guess I hadn't really believed it. Boy was I wrong. Because I was living it...

So believe it or not, I took my own advice. I'm going to take you on a little trip now. A trip into my own personal testimony about how I took the tips I wrote for you to implement, and I tried them myself. You have to understand I was about to give my husband the "let's separate" talk to see if things between us would get better. I was done. Really really done. Divorce seemed the only sensible solution. I felt like I didn't even know my own husband any more. And I just wanted to quit hurting because I really did miss him a lot.

It's Monday morning. No one is up yet. So I'm going to make a plan to give him what I know he likes. Tonight I'm going to get to bed and wear a favorite piece of lingerie. And see if that works for anything. I know it's only one night. So I will try tomorrow night too.

Well last night did and did not go as planned. I couldn't bring myself to put on a piece of lingerie. I wasn't feeling it if you know what I mean. So I lied down in bed next to my husband and felt like I was as far away as Mars. Yes the planet. That's pretty far, isn't it? It seemed like another night of disaster was inevitable. I think he felt like that too. But we did what we could to salvage the night. And began talking about 'us'.

Through talking we identified some things we had been missing over the past few months. The time we spent together was getting shortened. Instead of coming home for lunch break, he had chosen to work through lunch to net us about $150.00 extra each week. Which was a joint decision. Also, he had been spending extra time after work helping his mom move. And to top it all off, an injury I had sustained while running left us unable to go to the gym, a time when we used to be alone together. We refer to it as our 'relationship bank'. We were only making withdraws and no deposits. So we did something totally insane (well at least for us with 5 kids still in the home). We arranged for an overnight babysitter and scheduled a hotel room stay 6 weeks in the future.

But what about now? That certainly didn't fix now. And honestly if we waited until then, I feared there wouldn't be any 'us' left to fix. I was angry, I was bitter. I resented the fact that we had allowed our marriage to slip away. Then I fell asleep. Yes, that's right…I fell ASLEEP.

I'm sure my husband was still talking but was unaware of my slipping away. I woke up, and then fell back into unconsciousness. What the heck was wrong with me? Sleeping wasn't going to fix anything. Yet, I couldn't stay awake no matter how hard I tried. My sex drive was asleep too.

I woke up once more and struggled to keep my eyes open. And then, something amazing happened. I started to caress my husband's stomach. I usually waited for him to touch me. But this time I guess because I was half asleep I was feeling frisky. Or maybe I was too tired to be fully aware of what I was doing. Well, either way caressing was apparently exactly what he needed and it was exactly what we needed to solve this problem.

Caressing him, I moved down into ummm other areas. And then after a few minutes I just leaped on top of him and let nature take its course. Sex was wonderful, although rather quick. Both of us ended satisfied. And all of a sudden, I felt connected to my husband again. It was definitely an AHA moment.

You see, both of us were feeling the vast space that we had allowed to enter between us. Because we hadn't put up a schedule for romance, time together, etc…life had slowly caved in and consumed practically all of our alone time. To the point where neither one of us was willing to give to the other. If we had stuck to our scheduled times together…like date nights out, date nights in, gym time, lunch time, etc…this issue wouldn't have unearthed its ugly head. But we hadn't been checking our time together at all. And so we devised a plan to help repair our brokenness.

First, we scheduled an overnight hotel stay and arranged an overnight sitter. Oh yes we did. Finally. After all this time we were actually going to get away for the night without any children. This really gave me something to look forward to. Then, we scheduled our next night out and arranged for a neighbor to pop over and babysit for a few hours. It was the best $20.00 we'd spent in a while. Yes, we give $10.00 an hour. That is fair to give to any teenager. Any more than that and you won't be able to afford dinner when you go out...at least we won't.

But this didn't solve our issue. We still had fights, we still wanted to quit, and we still weren't connecting. But it was a plan. And we just stuck to it and decided that we would try hard to make it work. Repairing your relationship may not be a one-time event. Chances are it is going to take several weeks to fix the brokenness. And during that time you both will have to make sacrifices. But why take it so seriously? Well, you have to because being parents of twins has statistically proven you are at a higher risk of divorcing. Check out the conclusion of one scientific study...

"Twins at first birth were associated with greater parental divorce compared to singletons (OR 1.08, 95% CI 1.01–1.16; absolute risk 13.7% with twins vs 12.7%, $p = 0.02$). The association was statistically greater among mothers not attending college (14.9% with twins vs 13.3%, $p = 0.01$) compared to those with some college (10.4% with twins vs 10.5%, $p = 0.34$); those with children older than 8 years (15.6% with twins vs 13.5%, $p < 0.01$) compared to younger children (10.6% with twins vs 10.8%, $p = 0.42$); and those with at least one twin girl (13.8% with twins vs 12.6%, $p = 0.03$) compared to twin boys (12.1% with twins vs 12.5%, $p = 0.38$).

Mothers with four or more children had a larger association between birth of twins and divorce (15.4% for mothers with twins at fourth birth vs 11.3% for all other mothers with four or more children, $p < 0.01$) compared to mothers with twins at first through third births (13.7% for twins at first birth vs 12.7%, $p = 0.02$)."

Source

WRAP UP

I really want to thank you for taking the time to read this book. I worked on it for over 2 years because, quite frankly, I was extremely busy with my twins. So this last section I'd like to leave you with some encouragement. And some last minute instructions.

Please take time for yourself every day. Don't forget that mom needs to be healthy and strong for her family. As you are out raising these unique individuals, don't lose sight of how unique YOU are because you've been given this opportunity that not many other women get to experience. As difficult as the road is ahead of you, it ends at a wonderful place. Those moments daily that you get to experience with your twins will last through a lifetime. The understanding that you gain about life, and the strength you receive as you conquer each day is world changing. And as we travel full throttle into the 21st Century, the importance twins play in forming our future grows with every passing moment.

Just recently companies have begun to study twins to prove the worth of their products. And science has just begun to embrace the value of placing identical twins on two different groups of the same research studies. The answers to many of life's problems, and the solutions to many of science's questions, have been in existence since creation. We were all just looking in the wrong places. Twins are the solution. Twins are the answers, to many of the questions. Isn't it exciting that you get to help raise these wonder humans? So enjoy the journey. Take good care of yourself. Eat healthy, exercise, and learn to take care of the little things for you too. For the answer to the cure for cancer may be sitting in your living room eating you out of house and home!

God bless you and now go enjoy your twins!

RESOURCES FOR SUCCESS

This is the section where I've included all lists that you can make copies of to help you on your road to success.

Scroll to next page for first chart!

RELATIONSHIP CHARTS

Ways to trigger fear in women. Men, do not ever…

1. Boss her around by telling her what to do.
2. Being short with her.
3. Neglect her by ignoring her.
4. Ignore her feelings.
5. Give the cold shoulder.
6. Take her for granted.
7. Limit her spending critically instead of making financial decisions together.
8. Tell her to stop worrying, to get over it, and tell her she's making a big deal out of nothing.
9. Letting her know that she talks too much.
10. Saying anything negative about her weight.
11. Pout.
12. Shut down or totally withdraw.
13. Threaten to quit your job.
14. Become flirty with other women. Even friend's wives or "taken" women.
15. Look at other women for more than a glance. Even on the television this can trigger a long battle for the two of you.
16. Tell her she's just like her mom.
17. Complain to her about her girlfriends.
18. Don't listen to her ideas.
19. Buy a sports car/motorcycle for yourself.

Ways to trigger fear in a man. Women, do not ever...

1. Correct what he says.
2. Question his judgment or lack or judgment.
3. Don't include him and consult him in important decisions.
4. Keep him from doing things to help you out.
5. Make him feel inadequate.
6. Overreact, yes even on PMS days you must try to stay calm   around him.
7. Ignore what his desires are.
8. Focus and complain about what you don't have or didn't get.
9. Withhold praise from him.
10. Speak to him using a harsh tone.
11. Be spontaneous and spring things on him abruptly (unless it's a surprise date).
12. Undermine his authority, especially in front of the kids.
13. Use condescending tones.
14. Criticize his personality.
15. Complain about his job.
16. Show little interest in what he is interested in.
17. Criticize his family no matter how crazy they are.
18. Make comparisons to other men, especially exes.
19. Focus on your state of unhappiness.
20. Value friends before him. Put friends first.

FREE HOME DATE NIGHT IDEAS

Rent a movie and watch it in bed

Get up early and eat breakfast together

Camp in the backyard

Candlelight shower

Candlelight dinner

Ice cream date night on the porch

Enjoy cocktails or non-alcoholic cocktails together

Split a dessert

Fireplace camp out

Snuggle to a movie in the living room

Have a picnic in front of the television

Theme night

Game night

Dance the night away

Workout together

BODY BY BELINDA

Meal 1 (breakfast)
3 hard boiled eggs (remove the yolk from two of the eggs)
1/2 cup cooked oatmeal OR
1 cup of brown rice OR
1 cup cream of wheat
10 almonds

(THIS NUTRITIONAL PLAN IS DESIGNED TO REMOVE PROCESSED FOODS BECAUSE THEY ARE LOADED WITH CHEMICALS THAT MAY ACTUALLY INHIBIT THE WEIGHT LOSS PROCESS) THEREFORE THE FIRST 2 WEEKS WILL INCLUDE NO PACKAGED FOODS LIKE CEREAL OR PROTEIN BARS

Meal 2 (BELINDA'S FAVORITE SNACK)
Small apple
1 tablespoon of natural peanut butter (level tablespoon NOT heaping ☺)

Meal 3
Chicken breast (3 or 4 oz)
1 cup of green beans
1 small sweet potato or small red potato

Meal 4
1/2 grapefruit
20 almonds

Meal 5

Lean protein (chicken, fish, sirloin, London broil)
Salad with oil and vinegar (try not to use packaged salad dressing if you do look for dressing without msg or chemicals of this nature) OR
2 cups green veggies like green beans or asparagus (this is a natural diuretic)

After dinner snack if must have something
AIR POPPED POPCORN FROM KERNELS NOT THE MICROWAVE STUFF OR
1 CUP OF GREEK YOGURT

AFTER TWO WEEKS OF PREVIOUS DIET

Meal 1 (breakfast)

3 hard boiled eggs (remove the yolk from two of the eggs) OR
Scrambled eggs whites prepared with non-stick spray OR
1 Cup Low-fat (2% or 1%) cottage cheese OR
1 Cup of Greek Yogurt
2 slices of whole wheat toast plain or with small amount of light Smart Balance spread OR
1 Serving of High Fiber Cereal
1/2 cup cooked oatmeal OR
1 cup of brown rice OR
1 cup cream of wheat
10 almonds

Meal 2

1 Serving of fruit
1 tablespoon of natural peanut butter (level tablespoon NOT heaping ☺) OR
Mozzarella cheese stick

Meal 3
Lean protein (chicken, fish, sirloin, London broil 3 or 4 oz)
1 cup of green beans or small salad
1 small sweet potato or small red potato OR serving of brown rice

Meal 4
1 Serving of Fruit
20 almonds

Meal 5
Lean protein (chicken, fish, sirloin, London broil)
Salad with oil and vinegar OR
2 cups green veggies like green beans, broccoli, or asparagus

After dinner snack if must have something
AIR POPPED POPCORN FROM KERNELS NOT THE MICROWAVE STUFF OR
1 CUP OF GREEK YOGURT

*For one of the above meals you can supplement with a protein shake but make sure it's pure protein without any added sweeteners and not a lot of ingredients (purchase this at the health food store) and mix it with 8 oz. skim milk.

EXERCISE CHARTS

Activity (1-hour duration) Weight of person and calories burned (chart taken from mayoClinic.com)

	160 lbs(73 kg)	200 lbs(91 kg)	240 lbs(109 kg)
Aerobics, high impact	533	664	796
Aerobics, low impact	365	455	545
Aerobics, water	402	501	600
Backpacking	511	637	763
Basketball game	584	728	872
Bicycling, < 10 mph, leisure	292	364	436
Bowling	219	273	327
Canoeing	256	319	382
Dancing, ballroom	219	273	327
Football, touch or flag	584	728	872
Golfing, carrying clubs	314	391	469
Hiking	438	546	654
Ice skating	511	637	763
Racquetball	511	637	763
Resistance training	365	455	545

Rollerblading
548	683	818

Rope jumping
861	1,074	1,286

Rowing, stationary
438	546	654

Running, 5 mph
606	755	905

Running, 8 mph
861	1,074	1,286

Skiing, cross-country
496	619	741

Skiing, downhill
314	391	469

Skiing, water
438	546	654

Softball or baseball
365	455	545

Stair treadmill
657	819	981

Swimming, laps
423	528	632

Tae kwon do
752	937	1,123

Tai chi
219	273	327

Tennis, singles
584	728	872

Volleyball
292	364	436

Walking, 2 mph
204	255	305

Walking, 3.5 mph
314	391	469

Workout

<u>Squat</u>-*2 sets of 10-12. Progress to 4 sets of 15*
Description-
Stand with feet about hip distance apart and parallel. Feet should be lined up with your shoulders. Dumbbells should be at your sides.
Bend at knees and stick glutes out behind you.
Keep back straight and the weight in your heels as you lower towards ground, mimicking sitting in a chair, arms at sides.
Sometimes it's helpful if you do squats in front of a chair.
As you return to fully standing, squeeze your glutes.
Progress to Squat Press
Same motion as above, but as you return to fully standing and squeeze your glutes, take dumbbels at shoulders and press towards the ceiling. Return back to shoulders to repeat entire movement.

<u>Deadlift</u>-*2 sets of 10-12. Progress to 4 sets of 15*
Description-
Stand with feet hip distance apart and parallel as you did with the squat.
With straight legs and back, hinge at hips while reaching arms down toward floor.
The dumbbells should be in front of your shins at bottom of movement. If that hurts at all in the back, only lower the weights to knee height.
Return to starting position by squeezing glutes.
Progress to Deadlift Row
Same motion as above, but as you bring the dumbbells to bottom of the movement, then engage your back and pull the dumbbells up by squeezing your shoulder blades together and rowing back with your elbows. Return to bottom of deadlift exercise and then return to starting position by squeezing glutes.

Bicep Curls-*2 sets of 10-12. Progress to 4 sets of 10-12*

Description-
Stand with feet shoulder width apart and parallel.
With dumbbells in hands, arms at sides, palms up
Lift weights up by bending elbows and squeezing biceps.
Keep elbows tucked into sides.
Return to start and repeat.

Progress to Curl Press
As you squeeze biceps and keep elbows tucked into sides, rotate your hands to point palms in front of you and away. Keep abs tight as you now press dumbbells up towards ceiling. Return weights to about shoulder height, rotate to face palms towards you.
Return to start position and repeat.

Overhead Dumbbell Presses-*2 sets of 10-12. Progress to 4 sets of 10-12*

Description
Stand with feet hip distance apart and parallel, abs drawn in.
With dumbbells in hands, arms bent out to sides at 90-degree angle with knuckles up, hands at shoulders.
Press weights overhead, keeping abs tight.
Lower weights slowly and return to start position and repeat.

Progress to Overhead Dumbbell Press standing on one leg for Balance during whole movement. Switch leg that you stand on for each set
While doing above exercise, stand on one foot with other foot placed near ground. Remain on one foot through entire set. Switch standing foot for each set.
Progress to keeping foot towards knee with knee and hip bent.

Triceps Extension, right arm then left arm-*2 Sets of 10-12. Progress to 4 sets of 10-12*
Description

Stand with feet shoulder width apart, right hand on hip
Reach left arm straight up holding dumbbell
Bend arm at elbow and drop weight slowly to just before 90 degrees
Squeeze tricep to slowly straighten back up.
Repeat on left arm for full set then switch to right arm. Once you complete both sides you have completed one set.

Progress to Tricep Dips off Couch or Bench

Stand in front of couch or bench facing away.
Place your hands on front edge of couch or bench.
Slowly lower yourself down in a sitting position until you've reached a 90-degree bend in elbows.
Press yourself back up through the triceps until your elbows extend almost fully.
To make this movement easier, bring your feet closer to the couch or bench.
To make this movement more challenging, bring your feet further out from the couch or bench.

Assisted Push Ups-*2 Sets of 10 reps. Progress to 3 sets of 12 reps*

With body facing floor bend at knees place hands on floor in line with shoulders.
Squeeze your back slightly to stabilize your shoulders.
Assuming a nice push up position with abs held in forming a straight line from knees to shoulders (at an angle) bend at elbows bringing your chest towards the floor.
When you get close to the floor, push back up using your chest.
Return to beginning and repeat.

Progress to Regular Push Ups

Same movement as above but place feet on floor instead of knees.

Dumbbell Back Rows-*2 Sets of 10 reps. Progress to 4 sets of 15 reps*

Stand hinged forward at hip, keeping back straight and abs pulled in.

Bring dumbbells to your sides, reaching to the floor.

Bend at elbows to pull weights up toward chest, squeeze shoulder blades together as you bring weights back in a rowing manner.

Return to beginning and repeat. This movement should be slow and controlled throughout.

ABS

Plank *First hold for 5 seconds 12 reps. Progress to more time holding and less reps to eventually get to 60 second holds 3 reps with 1-minute rest in between.*

Lie face down

Push up off floor onto elbows and toes. Keep elbows in line with your shoulders.

Keeping a straight line, hold the position with a flat back throughout the exercise.

Slowly lower yourself to ground, rest, and repeat.

Hip Bridge-*As many as you can do for 60 seconds at least 2 second hold in top of movement.*

Description-

Lie on your back on a mat on the floor.

Place both hands by sides, knees bent.

Keep weight in heels, squeeze glutes and push hips up towards ceiling so body is in one line from knees to shoulders.

Return to starting position and repeat.

Reverse Curls-*2 Sets of 20. Progress to as many as you can do!*

Lie on floor on back with both hands behind head.

With legs bent, pull knees in towards head.

Movement should be minimal, only a few inches.

Return to start and repeat.
Progress the movement by lifting shoulders off floor into a crunch and hold throughout the movement.

Basic Crunch-2 Sets of 20. Progress to as many as you can do!
Lie on floor on back with both hands behind head. Knees bent.
Keep lower back on floor.
Lift shoulders off floor, engaging your core muscles.
Return to start and repeat.
This move can be done at same time as reverse curls to make it more difficult.

Right Oblique Crunch-1 Set of 15. Progress to 2 sets of 12 reps
Lie on floor on back with right hand behind head. Knees bent.
Place left hand on right side of stomach.
Lift right shoulder off floor.
Bring right elbow towards left knee.
Return to start and repeat.

Left Oblique Crunch-1 Set of 15. Progress to 2 sets of 12 reps
Lie on floor on back with left hand behind head. Knees bent.
Place right hand on left side of stomach.
Lift left shoulder off floor.
Bring left elbow towards right knee.
Return to start and repeat.

Crossover Crunch-1 Set of 15. Progress to 2 sets of 12 reps
Lie on floor with both hands behind head, knees bent.
Lift right shoulder off floor and lift leg off floor.
Bring right elbow to left knee.

Repeat on other side and alternate the movement.

Superman-*1 Set of 10 reps. Progress to 3 sets of 12 reps*

Lie face down on your stomach with arms and legs extended. Keep your neck in a neutral position.

Keeping your arms and legs straight but not locked and torso stationary, lift your arms and legs up toward the ceiling to form an elongated "u" shape with your body. Back should arch up and arms and legs should lift off the floor.

Hold for 2 to 5 seconds and then lower back down to starting position.

Repeat.

REFERENCES

Gillicirist, Adam . Hormonal Imbalance in Women During Pregnancy. July 7, 2011 Eastern Drugs.com
http://www.easterndrugs.com/blog/human-body/hormonal-imbalance-in-women accessed by the Internet December 22, 2012

Jena, Anupam, Goldman, Dana, Joyce, Jeffrey *Association Between the Birth of Twins and Parental Divorce*. April 1, 2012 National Center for Biotechnology Information. National Institute of Health.com
http://www.ncbi.nlm.nih.gov/pmc/articles
/PMC3069855/ accessed by the Internet September 28, 2014

Maloni, J., Suen, L. & Wang, K. (2002). Dysphoria among hospitalized high-risk pregnant women hospitalized with antepartum bed rest: A longitudinal study. Nursing Research, 51(2), 92-99.

Mayo Clinic *Exercise for Weight Loss. Calories Burned in One Hour.* http://www.mayoclinic.com/health/exercise/SM00109 accessed by the Internet 12/14/2012

U.S. Food and Drug Administration – Dietary Supplements.
http://www.fda.gov/food/dietarysupplements/default.htm accessed by the Internet 11/08/2012

Special thanks to Jodi Barnett Hamm, Belinda Ann Hope, Robyn Rinberger, and my husband Bill Powell for the contributions they've provided for this book. Without your help I would not have been able to finish it. Thank you so much from the bottom of my heart.

www.ingramcontent.com/pod-product-compliance
Lightning Source LLC
Chambersburg PA
CBHW070642290526
45790CB00001B/167